HOW DOES HOMEOPATHY WORK?

Homeopathy is based on the principle of using minute amounts of a remedy that in large quantities would cause the symptoms of the ailment being treated. For example, the same agent in an onion that causes the running nose and burning eyes in a healthy person might be used to stimulate the body's defenses against those symptoms in a hay fever sufferer.

This easy-to-follow handbook shows you how to work with your body's natural defense mechanisms to treat acute problems such as injuries and infections. Clear, detailed diagnostic charts guide you through the selection of appropriate remedies, while simple instructions help you achieve better health through a natural, holistic approach.

HOMEOPATHY

by Beth MacEoin

HarperPaperbacks
A Division of HarperCollins*Publishers*

HarperPaperbacks   *A Division of* HarperCollins*Publishers*
10 East 53rd Street, New York, N.Y. 10022

Copyright © 1992, 1994 by Beth MacEoin
All rights reserved. No part of this book may be used or reproduced in any manner whatsoever without written permission of the publisher, except in the case of brief quotations embodied in critical articles and reviews. For information address Hodder & Stoughton Ltd., Mill Road, Dunton Green, Sevenoaks, Kent, England. Further details may be obtained from the Copyright Licensing Agency Limited, 90 Tottenham Court Road, London WIP 9HE, England.

This book was published in Britain in 1992 by Hodder & Stoughton Ltd., as part of the Headway Lifeguides Series.

First HarperPaperbacks printing: October 1994

Printed in the United States of America

HarperPaperbacks and colophon are trademarks of HarperCollins*Publishers*

❖ 10 9 8 7 6 5 4 3 2 1

For Denis, without whose patience, love, and encouragement this book would never have been written.

Contents

Acknowledgments

My warmest thanks are due to many people who have offered help and advice with this project. At the earliest stage my agent, Teresa Chris, offered immensely practical help and encouragement, for which I shall always be grateful to her. Karen Solem has also been extremely enthusiastic and supportive in her capacity as editor of the updated American text.

Thanks must be extended to Stephen Gordon, who has been especially helpful in offering advice on the more technical aspects of this manuscript. I am also deeply indebted to John Morgan and Angela Morse; the latter must also be thanked, not only for her incisive comments and advice on the text of this book, but for initially encouraging in me a love of this subject. Rima Handley must also not be forgotten for having taken time out from an already extremely busy schedule to read the manuscript. Thanks must also be extended to Dana Ullman and Dr. Stephen Cummings, whose book on the same subject entitled *Everybody's Guide to Homeopathic Medicines: Taking Care of Yourself and Your Family with Safe and Effective Remedies* provided me with inspiration, and some very practical advice on the nuts and bolts of first aid. Dana Ullman has also been especially helpful in giving sound and practical advice on changes that have been made to make the text relevant to an American audience.

My mother Nancy must also be thanked for keeping the household sane while I have been occupied with writing this book. Finally, the largest measure of thanks must go to Denis, Daniel, and Jonathan. Without their unwavering vision and enthusiasm for this project, I would have given up in despair and impatience many times.

Foreword

Prior to the epidemic of AIDS, the general public and even many physicians had little sense of the importance of the body's immune system. The subject was too intangible for most people, in part because the immune system was not directly created by a specific organ or gland but was a more holistic response of the body.

Such has been the problem with homeopathic medicine. Because homeopaths must individualize a remedy to a person, instead of giving the same medicine to everyone, homeopathy has a similar intangibility. The exceedingly small doses that homeopaths use have simply exacerbated homeopathy's problem; but careful observation of the long-term effects of conventional drugs and the action of homeopathic medicines helps make more tangible the value of the latter.

Although powerful drugs may effectively inhibit symptoms, they usually do not elicit a true cure, and rather than stimulating the body's immune system, tend to suppress it. On the other hand, instead of overwhelming the body, individually prescribed homeopathic medicines catalyze it to heal itself, rather than doing something to or for it. The small doses used in homeopathy may actually be the most powerful pharmacological agents to augment the body's immune and defense system.

Dr. Emil Adolph von Behring, the father of immunology, directly acknowledged that immunizations and homeopathic medicine derived in part from a similar conceptual basis. Ironically, it was in 1796, the very year that Edward Jenner did his first experiments with the cowpox vaccine as a way to prevent smallpox, that Dr.

Samuel Hahnemann did the first experiments that led to the development of homeopathic medicine.

Jenner's immunizations were more readily accepted than Hahnemann's discovery, largely because the former's contribution fitted the emerging industrial revolution's assembly-line type of thinking. Like a cog in the wheel, every person on the medical assembly-line was given the same medicine. Hahnemann's emphasis on individualizing a medicine to the person, not the disease, did not fit that day's model of thinking or practice.

Now that modern physiology has taught us that there is a connection between mind and body and that each person responds individually and uniquely to a disease, the basic holistic principles of homeopathic medicine and its individualized approach are making more sense.

As homeopathy begins to make more sense to greater numbers of people, user-friendly books that teach people how to individualize a homeopathic medicine to a sick person will become increasingly important. Beth MacEoin's new book on homeopathy provides practical charts that greatly simplify the process of individualizing a homeopathic medicine.

Using homeopathic medicines for self-care and family care is empowering. Not only do the remedies work very effectively, they empower people by aiding them to help themselves in a simple and practical way.

This book is a good first step in learning how to use homeopathic medicines. The next step is yours: use this book, and you will be healthier for it.

Dana Ullman, M.P.H.
Author of *Discovering Homeopathy* and *Homeopathic Medicines for Children and Infants* and co-author of *Everybody's Guide to Homeopathic Medicines*. Berkeley, CA.

Introduction

This book is intended as a basic introduction to homeopathy for the person who knows nothing about the subject, as well as providing a very practical self-care handbook that may be used for those conditions that may be safely managed at home. As always in a book of this kind, very firm guidelines are given about when to call for professional help, and symptoms that indicate you are likely to be getting out of your depth are highlighted. (In severe emergencies, your first port of call should, of course, be your family practitioner or the emergency room of your local hospital. In less pressing circumstances, patients should contact their family practitioner initially; when the immediate emergency has been taken care of, they may consider finding a competent homeopath to investigate the problem more deeply.) However, I am sure you will find judicious homeopathic prescribing within this framework a rewarding, exciting, and enjoyable experience, even if the challenge seems rather daunting at first.

The information in this book is advisory in nature and should not be regarded as replacing the services of a physician. If in doubt, consult a medical professional. Neither the publishers nor the author accept responsibility for the consequences of self-treatment.

WHAT IS HOMEOPATHIC MEDICINE?

Homeopathic medicine is a system of healing that has been in existence for almost two hundred years. It is practiced by both conventional doctors and professional homeopaths on a worldwide basis. In expert hands, homeopathy provides a way of restoring the sick individual to good health in a gentle, thorough, and effective manner.

The Concept of Similars

The word *homeopathy* comes from the Greek, and may be translated as "similar suffering." In other words, the agent which can cause disease in a well person may be used to therapeutic advantage in the person who is sick and whose symptoms resemble those of the agent. This was a concept that had existed from the time of Hippocrates, but Samuel Hahnemann, the originator of homeopathy as a modern medical theory, took the basic idea much further by developing it into a full therapeutic system. In doing so, he put forward a theory of health and disease that ran completely opposite to the medical thinking of his own day and ours (this latter generally referred to as *allopathy*). Instead of prescribing a drug that would oppose the symptoms of illness and suppress them, Hahnemann advocated the use of a medicinal substance that worked with the body and encouraged it to throw off the symptoms by stimulating it to work more effectively.

"Provings" of Remedies

In order to find out the effects a medicinal substance would have on an individual in good health, Hahnemann carried out a series of controlled experiments on himself and other volunteers. Those experiments he called "provings"; they involve taking small amounts of a substance repeatedly and recording the effects. The people selected must be in good health and ready to observe and record in meticulous detail any changes in their emotional or physical health during the period of the experiment. Today many hundreds of homeopathic medicines are in use that have been proved in just this manner, and the process continues as new medicines are introduced.

The Single Dose

When treating patients with chronic health problems, homeopathic practitioners will usually give a single dose of the indicated medicine. Reactions to that dose are then observed, and a decision is made whether to wait longer, give a second dose (of the same or greater strength), or change the remedy altogether.

One of the main arguments in favor of administering medicines one dose at a time is that it is very difficult to determine how effective a particular remedy has been if it is closely followed by, or even mixed with another. However, there are homeopaths who would argue that combination formulas (a mixture of three to eight homeopathic medicines in a low potency) have a place in acute prescribing, especially in situations where individualizing characteristics are very hard to find. It should be stressed that chronic conditions such as eczema, asthma, or hay fever will need professional treatment from a qualified homeopath, since neither a combination formula nor an individually selected acute remedy is likely to be able to deal with a deep-seated predisposition to the condition. For a cure to take place, the skill, training, and professional judgment of a homeopathic practitioner is needed to select the indicated remedy and evaluate the progress of the case, deciding when to wait, and when to repeat or change the indicated remedy.

The Minimum Dose

Parallel with the notion of treating by similars, Hahnemann also developed the theory that the dose of the medicine administered should be the smallest possible to effect a cure. This appears to have been a preoccupation of his from the time he spent in practice as an orthodox physician, during which he was increasingly appalled by the side-effects he witnessed as a result of allopathic treatment. He therefore experimented using smaller and smaller doses of medicinal substances, until he came to a point of dilution where orthodox science parted company with him. Although at this level of dilution, no molecules of the original substance could be found, Hahnemann found that these highly dilute medicines had a profound effect in stimulating the process of healing in the body, provided they went through an additional process of vigorous shaking or *succussion* at each stage of dilution. In fact, he found that the higher the dilution and the further away he got from the material dose, the stronger the medicinal effect proved to be—as long as the similarity between the medicine and the patient's state still existed.

It must be emphasized that for a substance to be homeopathically active, the twin processes of dilution and succussion must both be carried out; the dilution alone is not enough to render the remedy medicinally useful.

The Importance of the Individuality of the Sick Person

In homeopathic practice, each sick person is seen as an individual who will respond to ill health in his or her own particular way. A note is made of any changes from the patient's normal condition on the physical, mental, and emotional levels: it is the analysis of this vital information that will lead to the selection of the most appropriate homeopathic medicine.

If we take an example of two people suffering from the common cold, we are likely to find that they share common symptoms of nasal discharge, sore throat, and a cough. This information in its general sense will do nothing to lead us to the appropriate homeopathic medicine, because it conveys nothing of the way the individual is expressing his or her illness.

In order to discover this, we need to inquire far more deeply into the individual characteristics of the symptoms to establish a sharper picture. Upon closer questioning we may discover that one person complains of a scanty, clear, burning nasal discharge, while the other has a profuse, yellowy-green, thick and bland secretion. The first person has been unbearably chilly since catching the cold and feels happiest hugging the fire, while the other also feels chilly but is generally much worse in stuffy rooms and better getting fresh air. Our chilly individual with the nasal discharge that burns the nostrils may also have noticed since the onset of the cold that she has felt unusually anxious, restless, and fussy and has a cough that is very dry and troublesome at night. On the other hand, the sufferer with the aversion to stuffy rooms and the multi-colored mucous may complain of feeling very weepy and in need of sympathy since the cold came on, and find that he has a very productive cough that is particularly loose in the mornings.

If we consider these two individuals in the light of the information given above, we see immediately how each one is expressing symptoms of illness in their own individual way. Therefore, one would not give the same homeopathic remedy to both, since their symptoms are not at all similar beyond the most general level, and it is the specifics that we are interested in. So we would suggest Arsenicum album in the first case, and Pulsatilla in the second. This is because the sick individual is being prescribed for, not the disease category in isolation.

HOW DOES HOMEOPATHY DIFFER FROM ORTHODOX MEDICINE?

In order to grasp fully the degree of contrast between the homeopathic and orthodox medical approaches to ill health, it is necessary to consider the context within which Samuel Hahnemann developed his own ideas.

Origins

Samuel Hahnemann was born in 1755 in Meissen and qualified as an orthodox doctor in 1779. The more he observed of orthodox treatments, the more alarmed he became at the appalling side-effects that patients were suffering. It is easy to forget how barbaric things were in medical practice as recently as the late eighteenth century. Patients were commonly subjected to treatment involving toxic substances like mercury in cases of venereal disease; bleeding practices were still much in vogue, including leeching, cupping, and venesection; and purging was often carried out to such a violent degree that patients were severely weakened.

By 1796, Hahnemann was so disturbed by what he had witnessed of current medicine that he decided to refrain from practicing as a physician and put his efforts instead into the translation of foreign medical texts. At the same time he conducted researches of his own into gentler ways of treating patients.

The major breakthrough came when he was translating Cullen's *Materia Medica*. Hahnemann was intrigued by Cullen's explanation for the effectiveness of quinine in treating cases of malaria but unsatisfied with his conclusion that it was the astringent properties of the substance that rendered it medicinally effective. Hahnemann decided that he would experiment by taking repeated doses of quinine himself and found that he began to develop symptoms of malaria, which went away once he stopped taking the medicine. As a result of this experiment, he began the long and tortuous path of developing the theory and practice of homeopathy: the treatment of sick individuals with similar substances rather than opposites. His clinical and theoretical work continued without interruption until his death in Paris in 1843.

After experimenting further along these lines with more medicinal substances, Hahnemann also began to work with more and more dilute forms of medicine, in an effort to promote the gentlest and most effective form of treatment. At this point, he made a quantum leap in his thinking: to the process of dilution, he added the systematic repetition of succussion or vigorous pounding. He found that both processes had to be carried out in order for a homeopathically prepared remedy to be medicinally effective. This process came to be called *potentization.*

The more he worked with patients using potentized medicines, the more he found that his observations ran counter to anything that could be explained by the scientific theory of his day. From the reactions he observed, the more dilute and succussed a substance became (even to the point where there was no molecule of the original substance left), the more potent the effect appeared to be on the sick person, always providing the "similarity" of the patient picture matched that of the remedy prescribed.

Concepts of Vital Energy

As Hahnemann continued to refine his ideas, he came to the conclusion that there must be some basic intelligence that governed the workings of the human body in good health. When this intelligence, or "vital force," came into conflict with a stressful stimulus that proved too strong for it to resist, symptoms of illness would be manifested in the person. These symptoms would be evidence of the body's own incomplete attempt to heal itself, thus providing clues as to the nature of the disturbance and essential information for the selection of the appropriate homeopathic medicine.

Looked at in this way, symptoms of illness acquire a more benign identity than they do from the perspective of orthodox medicine.

The Orthodox Medical Approach

Because modern medicine sees the human body as an object constantly under siege from hostile bacteria and viruses, many drug therapies work along the lines of searching for the "magic bullet" that will kill off the offending microbe. Unlike homeopathy, which attempts to stimulate the body's own defense mechanism to overcome an infection, orthodox medicine works by identifying the individual organism, in order to eliminate it with the appropriate drug.

The nature of the drugs used are also quite different in orthodox practice when compared to homeopathic selection of medicines. As we have previously pointed out, homeopathic remedies are selected because their effect on the human economy is similar to the body's own self-defense mechanism. They thus enable the body to fight the disease more effectively. Allopathic or orthodox drugs, however, work on a totally different basis, since they are chosen with the goal of countering the disease by producing an opposite effect. Everyday examples of these would include antacids to dilute overacidity in the stomach, laxatives to deal with constipation, and anti-inflammatories to dampen down inflammation. Because such drugs work by countering symptoms, patients often have to continue taking them on a long-term basis to keep the symptoms under control. The homeopathic approach is centered on helping the body work more efficiently so that it can throw off and overcome symptoms itself; consequently, the long-term aim of homeopathic treatment is to get the body sufficiently in balance so that medicinal intervention is unnecessary unless and until the body is again overwhelmed by stress.

COMMON PROBLEMS WITH THE ORTHODOX MEDICAL APPROACH TO HEALTH AND DISEASE

The Importance of the Whole Person

Unfortunately, because orthodox medical diagnosis puts so much emphasis on the common symptoms of disease in its selection of the appropriate drug therapy, it is easy to lose sight of the individual person in the pursuit of a diagnosis. As a result, people who are ill often feel that they have become primarily a walking case of whatever they are suffering from; a feeling that is often reinforced by the battery of investigative tests to which they may be subjected.

Because orthodox medicine seems to think of good health as the absence of disease rather than the positive acquiring of a healthy and well-regulated body, this has often led to people expecting a pill for every minor problem that arises. This is largely because doctors have lost sight of the human body as an entity that has a defense mechanism of its own, which, when healthy, can fight off transient illness itself. As a result, many people have lost touch with steps they can take to aid their body through short-term infections like the common cold. Sensible supportive measures such as keeping fluid intake high, a light and easily digested diet, avoiding extremes of heat and chill in the environment, and taking a few days rest are all likely to assist the body in its fight against infection. Unfortunately, many of us expect a magic pill to rid us of unpleasant symptoms, ignoring the messages our body is sending us that we may need to take it easy for a few days.

When homeopathy is used effectively, it is unlikely to abort symptoms of the common cold in their tracks, but it will support the body through the various stages so that the infection will pass more quickly and cause minimum complications. Because homeopathy is working to assist the body in its fight, any measures that can be taken to help the struggle will be supportive of homeopathic treatment. This is why in this book you will find extended sections in each chapter on general measures that can be taken in addition to prescribing homeopathic medicines.

Because homeopathic medicines are selected on the basis of matching the individual's symptom picture with the appropriate homeopathic remedy, any changes that have appeared in the individual since the onset of the illness will be worth noting. These changes are not restricted to any physical symptoms that have appeared, but also include emotional changes that may have surfaced since the illness commenced. It is very noticeable that people may experience any of the following reactions as a result of feeling unwell: tearfulness, irritability, excitability, withdrawal, or anxiety. Any change on this emotional level is as relevant to the selection of the appropriate homeopathic remedy as detailed information about aches and pains, nausea, mucous discharges, or fever.

There are some infections where orthodox medicine has little to offer in the way of drug therapy because the relevant agent has not been developed. Generally speaking, many viral infections are left to themselves because, with some exceptions, antiviral agents are not in broad use like antibiotics. Because the homeopathic approach is starting from a completely different premise of boosting the body's ability to overcome the infection, it is of little relevance whether the infection is of bacterial or viral origin. As a result, there are fewer limitations on the appropriate use of homeopathy for infectious illnesses.

HOW HOLISTIC IS HOMEOPATHY?

The term *holistic medicine* is one that many of us are very familiar with these days. Books have been devoted not only to the exploration of holistic therapies, but also to the wider concept of holistic living.

As concern with our external environment grows, and as that environment appears to be increasingly compromised by the excesses of a highly industrialized society, it is hardly surprising that many people are becoming concerned about how they set about achieving and protecting an optimum level of good health for themselves and their families. For such people, protecting the ecology of the individual body is becoming as pertinent an issue as protecting the rain forests, or defending the lives of whales.

Homeopathy is a system of healing that fits very well within this context, because of its concern with achieving and maintaining the integrity of the health of the individual person. Because the medicines used do not have the unpleasant side effects of more toxic drugs, they provide a gentle but extremely effective way of stimulating the body back to good health. Of course, homeopathy is not unique in occupying this position, since it has much in common with other therapies that one would broadly call holistic. These are therapies that also stress the need to get the individual person back to a state of good health rather than merely removing or suppressing symptoms. They include acupuncture, herbalism, ayurvedic medicine, chiropractic, and osteopathy.

Because homeopathy is genuinely concerned with the impact of the environment on the physical, emotional, and mental levels of the individual, you will find that homeopathic medicines are rarely selected on the basis of physical symptoms alone. There are, of course, some very straightforward first-aid situations where it would be needless to probe into the patient's state of emotional well-being. A sprained ankle or a bad bruise from a fall can be effectively prescribed for on the basis of detailed physical symptoms alone. Once one gets into the realm of stomach upsets, colds and flu, or transient anxiety states, however, any information about emotional changes may provide a vital clue to the selection of the appropriate remedy. If we go a step further and consider the homeopathic practitioner taking the case of a chronically sick individual, the question of the patient's emotional environment becomes even more crucial to the enterprise.

Who Can Benefit From Homeopathy?

Generally speaking, homeopathy is a system of medicine that is potentially helpful to anyone. Many homeopaths say that there are no barriers to homeopathy in treating diseases, but that there are some individuals who have more responsive defense mechanisms or immune systems than others.

Of course, there are serious diseases where the prognosis will be disheartening, and there will always be stubborn cases where response is slow in coming. If someone has suffered from an illness for many years and has undergone long courses of suppressive therapy, they are likely to find that they will take longer to respond than a young child who has recently fallen ill within the context of general good health.

Age is not a stumbling block to the suitability of homeopathy as a therapy: babies can be treated as effectively as the elderly. Homeopathy is also not limited to the treatment of humans: farm and domestic animals have been effectively helped by the use of veterinary homeopathy.

HOMEOPATHY IN THE UNITED STATES

The development of homeopathy in the United States is a fascinating subject. The American Institute of Homeopathy, founded in 1844, was the country's first national medical society. Two years later the American Medical Association was set up, and from this point until the early years of the twentieth century, the two organizations experienced an uneasy and acrimonious relationship.

As homeopathy gained ground in terms of popularity and success, conventional practitioners became increasingly unhappy. The success of homeopathy was based on extremely positive results in treating the various epidemic diseases that spread through Europe and America in the 1800s. It has been estimated that the death rate in homeopathic hospitals from these diseases was around fifty percent lower than that in conventional medical hospitals. During the cholera epidemic in Cincinnati in 1849, only three percent of homeopathic patients died, compared with between forty and sixty percent of those treated by conventional medical treatment.

Apart from these dramatic results in treating infectious illnesses, homeopaths were effective in treating a range of acute and chronic problems. The effectiveness of this treatment was acknowledged by some insurance companies, who offered a ten-percent discount to homeopathic patients because they tended to enjoy a longer life expectancy.

The quality of medical training given to homeopaths was of a very high standard and generally compared favorably with that of their orthodox colleagues. Homeopathic medical schools were set up in Boston University and the Universities of Michigan, Minnesota, and Iowa. Although acknowledged and accepted as a popular and viable alternative to orthodox medical treatment by patients, it is striking that this popularity is not acknowledged in accounts of the development of American medicine.

The fall of homeopathy was initiated by the Flexner Report of 1910, a nationwide survey of standards in medical education. Because the report favored a particular approach which emphasized the teaching of pathology and a physiochemical understanding of disease, and put great weight on the need for full-time teaching staff, homeopathic colleges were not rated highly. This was also because many of the lecturers did not devote themselves to teaching or research but remained in clinical practice. Many homeopathic colleges also included courses in pharmacology, a subject which the Flexner Report paid scant attention to.

In an attempt to come to terms with the findings of the Flexner Report, the syllabuses of homeopathic colleges were overstretched to accomodate pathology, chemistry, physiology, and other medical sciences. As a consequence, the teaching and practice of homeopathy began to suffer, with many homeopaths and patients losing interest. Other factors that also led to decline of homeopathic practice in America included improvements in sanitation, housing, food production, and the practice of conventional medicine. There was also the simple fact that homeopathy was more time-consuming and labor-intensive than ortho-dox medicine, due to the need to tailor each prescription to an individual patient. With the rise of the era of the "wonder drugs" in the first half of the twentieth century, it looked as though homeopathy was gone for good. However, as the legacy of these drugs — including unpleasant and often harmful side-effects and drug dependency — has gradually become apparent to the pub-lic, the study and practice of homeopathic medicine has undergone a renewal of interest and popularity.

In the United States today, the bulk of homeopathic practitioners are licensed professionals. It has been esti-mated that there are, in round figures, between 1,000 and 2,000 medical doctors, 750 naturopaths, 500 acupunctur-ists, 250 nurses, 250 dentists, and 500 veterinarians actively involved in the practice of homeopathy in America today. In addition, there are also an estimated two hundred lay practitioners in practice.

Although these numbers may seem insignificant in comparison with the popularity of homeopathy in countries such as India or in Europe, there is an observable increase of interest in homeopathy among American health professionals. Over the past two years the number of training programs has tripled, with introductory courses on offer at Harvard and at the Universities of Arizona, Virginia, Maryland, and California at San Francisco.

At present, there are three states that have separate homeopathic medical boards: these are Nevada, Arizona, and Connecticut. Although there are many homeopaths working as lay practitioners, these boards will only license medical doctors, but they do not state that homeopathic practice should be limited to the work of medical doctors within their respective states. There are also approximately nine states that have licensed naturopathic physicians who are legally permitted to prescribe homeopathic medicines for patients, and whose laws do not prevent homeopathic practice by others.

As the above information suggests, there is generally a lack of clarity in the United States regarding the legality of the practice of homeopathy by lay practitioners and other health professionals. This will, no doubt, be clarified as patient demand increases, and increasing numbers of lay and conventional physicians and other health workers are trained to practice homeopathy.

For an up-to-date directory of homeopaths in North America, contact either the National Center for Homeopathy or Homeopathic Educational Services (see Homeopathic Resources).

HOMEOPATHY ABROAD

Homeopathy is well established in Britain, with patients having the freedom to select practitioners from two possible avenues of training. There are conventional doctors who have obtained additional postgraduate training in homeopathy. These may work in the National Health Service, at one of the homeopathic hospitals in the capacity of consultant, or in private practice.

There is also a growing number of homeopathic practitioners who have received a thorough grounding in homeopathic theory and practice at one of the many homeopathic colleges. These graduates are free to apply for inclusion on the Register of the Society of Homeopaths. Although the bulk of professional homeopaths work in a private capacity, legislative changes have now made it possible for a doctor at an NHS practice to call on the services of alternative practitioners, including homeopaths.

Homeopathy flourishes in India, where it has received official recognition as a separate medical system with a government-approved Central Homeopathic Council. Homeopathic treatment is widely available from 200,000 or more practitioners, of whom 70,000 are registered with state boards. India has the largest number of homeopathic hospitals, and training may be obtained from over one hundred colleges.

In France, one may obtain homeopathic medicines and treatment very easily from orthodox physicians who have taken additional training in homeopathy. It was estimated in a recent survey that approximately twenty-five percent of the French public have used homeopathic medicine, and that 11,000 doctors adopt it as a therapy.

Homeopathy also enjoys a high profile in Germany as well as in other countries where it is either well-established or gaining ground. These include Mexico, Argentina, Brazil, Australia, South Africa, New Zealand, Holland, and Greece. Homeopathy has also started to develop in Eastern Europe and Russia.

1

Practical Homeopathy

WHAT CONDITIONS ARE APPROPRIATE FOR SELF-CARE?

You will find that certain health problems are conspicuous by their absence from this book. If you want to find out how to self-prescribe for eczema, migraines, asthma, or menstrual problems, I'm afraid you will not find them listed in the self-help sections. The reason for this is quite simple, and lies in the contrast between acute and chronic forms of disease.

If a problem is classed as *acute*, this does not refer to the severity of the condition. It is a term that defines a self-limiting condition; in other words, one that will clear up of its own accord given the right conditions and enough time for the body to deal with it. Good examples of acute problems include colds, influenza, food poisoning, and childhood infectious illnesses. You will find that the conditions covered by this book generally fall into the acute category.

Chronic problems, unlike acutes, are much less likely to resolve themselves, no matter how much time and ample opportunity the body is given to recuperate. The general pattern of chronic illness is that of repeated flare-ups, which may go into remission for a time but will always tend to return. Good examples of chronic problems would include asthma, hay fever, eczema, psoriasis, and irritable bowel syndrome. It is true to say that some chronic conditions will give rise to acute exacerbations within the chronic condition, but these should not be confused with an acute problem that arises without the bedrock of a chronic problem.

Generally speaking, acute conditions respond well to self-help prescribing, but chronic problems need help from a qualified practitioner. Case management of chronic conditions can be complicated, and the training of a professional is required to steer the patient toward a state of improved health. This is especially true of the management of skin conditions, since homeopaths generally view a persistent skin eruption as indicative of a deeper, underlying, inherited disorder that needs to be dealt with before the whole person can enjoy improved health. If the skin condition is combined with the patient suffering from a more internal disorder such as asthma, very careful case management is needed to deal with the overall improvement of the case. In cases such as these, the practitioner needs to be prepared for any complications that may arise during treatment, and must constantly use his or her professional judgment to assess how the patient is progressing.

You will find that hay fever is the one chronic condition that has been included in this book. The reasoning behind this is simple: for many people, the symptoms of hay fever during the summer resemble closely those of the common cold. In this situation, finding a helpful homeopathic remedy can be as straightforward as selecting the most appropriate remedy for an acute bout of cold. You will notice, however, that a statement appears at the top of the hay fever table advising anyone suffering from hay fever to seek professional help. This is because acute prescribing will do nothing to alleviate the underlying problem, and relief will only be obtained on a short-term basis. If professional help is sought for the condition, results on a long-term basis are likely to be much more satisfactory.

The omission of any other conditions that may be defined as acutes have been made on the basis of personal judgment. Headaches, for example, do not appear, since it has been my experience that it can be very difficult for the beginner to differentiate between various sorts of head pain. In this sort of situation, where individualizing characteristics can be hard to isolate, results can be disappointing. This is a purely subjective opinion and does not mean that you will find headaches ommited from other homeopathic self-care manuals.

You will also find that there is a strong emphasis in each section on which symptoms indicate that you may be getting out of your depth and that you need a professional opinion. Never be hesitant about getting help if you suspect a condition could be serious: in this situation it is always most prudent to err on the cautious side.

How Do I Learn More About Homeopathic Self-Care?

I would strongly urge anyone who has bought this book to attend one of the many classes in homeopathic first aid or self-care that are held across the country. It has been my own experience that a book can teach one a great deal about the basics of self-prescribing, but inevitably there will always be questions in the reader's mind that may not be covered by the information in the book. Once you have become familiar with this book, attending a homeopathic self-care class will give you the opportunity to discuss issues with other beginners like yourself, and your questions can be answered by the practitioner who is running the class.

If you would like to obtain information about self-care

classes in your area I would suggest you contact the
National Center for Homeopathy or Homeopathic
Educational Services for information about one of the
many hundred homeopathic study groups (see
Homeopathic Resources, p. 159).

WHERE CAN I OBTAIN HOMEOPATHIC MEDICINES?

You will find that there are increasing outlets for the sale
of homeopathic medicines, as the demand for homeopathic treatment is growing. Your local health food store is a
good place to start looking for a stock of basic homeopathic medicines.

There are pharmacies that also manufacture and supply
homeopathic medicines who are happy to deal with telephone orders. If you require any medicines that are slightly obscure, you will need to order from this source.
Names and addresses of homeopathic pharmacies are
given in Homeopathic Resources at the end of this book.

You will find that you can obtain homeopathic
medicines in the form of large or small tablets, granules,
pilules, powders, or in liquid form as tinctures. Gels, ointments, and tinctures are also available for external use.

Potencies

Most of the homeopathic medicines that can be bought
over the counter come in either 6c or 30c potency. The *c*
refers to the method of dilution that has been employed—
in this case, the centesimal scale of dilution. You may also
come across remedies that have a *∂* or *x* after the number;
this refers to the decimal scale. In the centesimal form of
dilution, the original substance to be rendered homeopathically active is diluted in alcohol. One drop of this
dilution is taken and added to ninety-nine drops of dis-
tilled water or alcohol and vigorously shaken to give the

first potency. This process is repeated
ing one drop of the previous potency
ninety-nine drops of dilutant. The sam
for the decimal scale, but the proportion
of tincture to nine drops of alcohol or disti

HOW TO USE THIS BOOK

How Do I Decide Which Remedy To Choose?

In order to use this book most effectively to find the most appropriate homeopathic medicine, you will need to do the following:

1. Using a notebook and pencil, write down any symptoms you have noticed since the onset of illness. These may refer to subjective changes as well as observable symptoms such as paleness in a person who normally has a healthy complexion.
2. Do remember that you are only interested in any changes from the normal state of the sick person. In other words, if someone is normally chilly, you would not attribute any importance to this. If, however, this person complained of feeling flushed and hot since their illness, this would be a valid symptom, because it signifies a change from the normal state for that individual.
3. Once you have listed all the symptoms you regard as being important, isolate any that seem peculiar. For instance, fever without thirst, chilliness with aversion to heat, or nausea that is relieved by eating. These are important symptoms as they may clinch your choice of remedy.
4. Try to identify a characteristic or theme running through the symptoms. You may find dryness a major characteristic running through skin texture,

sensations in the throat, and bowel movements. When you have a major thread like this running through the symptoms you have a head start.

5. Inquire if there has been a precipitating factor before illness set in, such as exposure to cold winds, or several nights' disturbed sleep, or a severe fright or shock. This is always worth noting.

6. Establish what makes the patient feel generally better or worse. This can apply to things that relieve or aggravate specific symptoms, or that have a general systemic effect on the patient.

7. Always note any changes on the emotional level that have occurred since the illness set in. Weepiness in a normally cheerful individual or anxiety and restlessness in a normally relaxed person are always symptoms of value.

8. By now you should have a fairly long list of symptoms, which I would suggest you divide by putting under the headings CAUSATIVE FACTORS, GENERAL SYMPTOMS, and MODALITIES (things which make the patient generally feel better or worse).

9. Do remember that the GENERAL SYMPTOMS heading can have a very wide scope, refering to any changes from normal on both the physical and emotional levels.

10. Now turn to the appropriate table in the relevant section of the book. Look down the left-hand column entitled Type to see which category is likely to fit most closely the group of symptoms you have on paper. If there is a causative factor, this will help you a great deal at this stage. This column will also give you information about what stage of illness you may be thinking of; in other words, whether one is thinking about early onset or a more established stage.

11. If you have found the category you want, check the information given under the next column entitled General Indications and see how it corresponds to

the general symptoms you have noted. (Additional notes applicable to each remedy are listed in the Remedy column.) It is unlikely that you will find a perfect match between the two, so don't worry if you can't find all the symptoms you have noted. What you will need to assess is whether the most important elements of the general indications cover the symptoms you have seen as important. To give an example, one would not consider Belladonna for someone with a cold unless they were very hot, dry, and feverish, and the cold had developed quite suddenly. If someone had a cold that had taken a long time to develop; looked pale, sweaty, and withdrawn; and felt very chilly; then clearly Belladonna would not fit and one would look elsewhere for the appropriate remedy.

12. If you are unsure what symptoms represent the key features of a homeopathic remedy, turn to the section at the back of the book entitled Remedy Keynotes. These will give you a quick overview of the essential features running through each remedy.

13. If you feel satisfied that the match between the symptoms of your patient and the homeopathic remedy you are considering are close enough, look at the columns entitled Worse From and Better From. If you feel that these also apply in general to the sick person, then it looks like you have found the most appropriate remedy.

14. Remember, what you are looking for is the information that characterizes what is individual in the sick person's symptoms. Always try to find out what it is that makes that person's case of flu or food poisoning different from another's. Common symptoms such as vomiting, sore throat, or cough will not help you at all in your search for the appropriate homeopathic remedy. You must always try to define how these broad symptoms affect the individual in the

way they perceive pain, the color and texture of their discharges, and how these specific symptoms affect their systems as a whole.

15. You will observe that the same medicines appear under different sections. For instance, Pulsatilla appears in the tables for indigestion, coughs, colds, and chicken pox, while Arsenicum album will appear in tables for vomiting, anxiety, coughs, and influenza. By using these tables and the keynotes at the back of the book, I hope you will begin to grasp the concept of these being multifaceted medicines that cover a range of complaints in their own individual ways. As you become more familiar with their uses you will begin to appreciate how each remedy has individual characteristics of its own, just as the sick person manifests his or her own disease in a way that is particular to them.

How to Take Homeopathic Medicines

Homeopathic medicines are normally in tablet form, but topical treatments such as tinctures, low-alcohol or nonalcoholic solutions, lotions, ointments, and gels are also available for external application.

1. Tip out a single dose of your selected remedy (a single dose being one tablet) onto a clean spoon or into the cap of the bottle (if there is one).
2. Do not wash the tablets down with water but suck them as you would a sweet in a clean mouth. Bear in mind that "a clean mouth" does not involve cleaning your teeth before taking the remedy but refers more to the necessity of avoiding eating, drinking, or cleaning your teeth too close to taking your remedy. It's a good idea to try to leave half an hour either side of eating or drinking.

3. Some homeopaths strongly recommend that you avoid the use of tea, coffee, and peppermint, and the application of strong-smelling rubs involving camphor. These are some of the substances that are thought to interfere with the effective action of homeopathic medicines. I would suggest that it is a good idea to avoid these if you are beginning to use homeopathy, since it avoids an element of potential confusion if it looks like the remedy you have selected is not working.

4. Store remedies away from strong light, odors, or extreme variations of temperature. A fairly cool, dark place is usually most suitable. If your remedies are kept under these conditions they will remain active, since they do not have a short shelf life.

5. If you accidentally spill some tablets out of the bottle, do not put them back in but throw them away.

6. If you are giving the remedy to a small child who has difficulty sucking a tablet, you can crush the tablet between two clean spoons and put the powder under the tongue to be absorbed, or rub it along the gums.

How Often to Repeat the Remedy

1. Take your first dose of the indicated remedy (a single dose being one tablet). Wait for half an hour; if there is no change, repeat the remedy. You can repeat the dose for up to three doses at half-hourly intervals.

2. If you notice an improvement by the second or third dose, STOP taking the remedy. This is an indication your body is now doing the work for itself, and that continuing the remedy will not be necessary unless the symptoms begin to recur. Once again, as soon as you notice an improvement occurring, stop taking the remedy.

3. The repetition suggested above is the recommended dose for a condition of sudden and recent onset, as in the case of food poisoning. If, however, your condition has been building up over a few days and appears to be more stubborn, you are likely to respond more favorably to repetition of the appropriate remedy three or four times daily over a period of three to four days. As before, once improvement takes place, STOP taking the remedy.

4. If there is no improvement after waiting the suggested time, take another look at the appropriate table and see if another remedy may be more suitable. If one remedy hasn't worked, there is no problem of incompatibility of medicines in moving on to another that may be more effective. Because the remedies work at a submolecular level, there is no risk of any chemical residue being left in the tissues that might spark off a toxic reaction.

5. You will find that most health food shops and pharmacies now stock homeopathic medicines in either 6c or 30c strength. I would suggest that if the condition is fairly mild and of recent onset that you try the indicated remedy for you in 6c potency and move on to the 30c if you feel only marginal improvement with the lower dose. It would be appropriate to begin with a 12c (available from homeopathic pharmacies) or 30c potency if the condition has been of longer duration and the symptoms are more severe.

6. Homeopathic medicines are not designed to be taken on a long-term basis for acute (short-lived) disorders. If you feel that you need to take them on a daily basis to achieve the desired effect, the chances are that you need more long-term, "constitutional" treatment from a homeopathic practitioner.

7. Above all, if you are at all confused and feeling a bit lost, always **seek professional help**.

Do remember that it is the frequency of repetition of the remedy that determines the strength of action of the remedy rather than the size of the dose. In other words, if one gives one, two, or five tablets at the same time it still counts as a single dose of the remedy. If, however, one gave a single tablet to the patient every ten minutes for an hour, this would count as six doses, since the remedy is being administered repeatedly.

Which Remedies Should I Buy?

I'm afraid it is very difficult to be absolutely specific about the exact number of remedies needed in the average first-aid kit, since one person's needs will not be the same as another's. For instance, anyone with babies and young children in their family is likely to need a kit that features remedies that are especially useful for childhood problems, such as Chamomilla and Colocynthis. These are not so likely to be indicated or useful in the kit required by a couple without children.

However, I would suggest that the following list of remedies would provide a good starter kit for someone who needs to have a basic range of the most frequently indicated homeopathic medicines:

Aconitum
Arnica
Arsenicum album
Belladonna
Bryonia
Carbo veg.
Gelsemium
Hypericum
Ignatia
Nux vomica
Phosphorus

Pulsatilla
Rhus tox.

Once you have this basic range of remedies, I would suggest useful additions would include the following:

Apis
Chamomilla
Ferrum phos.
Hepar sulph.
Ipecac
Ledum
Lycopodium
Merc sol.
Lachesis
Ruta
Staphysagria
Veratrum album

In addition, I would also suggest you obtain the following ointments and tinctures for topical administration:

Calendula Tincture: To be used *diluted* (1 part tincture to 10 parts boiled, cooled water) on cuts and grazes.

Calendula Ointment or Gel: To be applied after Calendula tincture on cuts and grazes to ensure the wound remains free of infection, and to help speed healing of tissue.

Urtica Urens Tincture: To be *diluted* and applied to minor burns and scalds.

These are, of course, arbitrary lists and should in no way be considered exhaustive. There are many more "basic" homeopathic remedies, all of them useful, but the above should provide the beginner with a sound basis on which to build.

What Potency Should I Buy?

Once again, this is a rather difficult question to answer, since different situations often require different potencies of the appropriate homeopathic remedy. For an explanation of potencies and their range please see the section entitled Potencies on page 4. I would suggest that you initially buy your remedies in 6c potency, and supplement these with the same remedies in 12c and 30c later. Do not worry unduly about selecting the optimum potency in the early days: if you have selected the most appropriate homeopathic remedy, use either a 6c, 12c, or 30c, remembering that the 6c potency will require more frequent repetition than the higher potencies.

When prescribing for children the same basic principles apply as for adults. You should bear in mind that conditions often develop more quickly and violently in children than adults, and the chosen homeopathic remedy may need to be repeated frequently in order to maintain an improvement. If the selected remedy in a 6c potency seems to be only giving partial or short-lived relief, consider moving on to the same remedy in a 30c potency. As always, do not repeat the remedy while an improvement is holding, only if there are signs that the symptoms are returning. If you are at all concerned about the seriousness of your child's condition, always get professional advice.

2

Homeopathic First Aid

ACCIDENTS AND INJURIES

Most advice given to people who have sustained a non-life-threatening injury tends to be limited to suggestions about rest, judicious use of painkillers, and the employment of supports (such as putting a limb in plaster while healing is taking place). There is a basic acknowledgment that, given the best conditions, the body will heal traumatized tissue itself, and that this takes time. Clearly, injuries or accidents that are more life-threatening will call for more radical measures, such as emergency surgery and drugs; but even in these situations, once the emergency phase is over, time is acknowledged once again as the prime healing agent.

Homeopathic Medicines and Accidents and Injuries

Prescribing for accidents and injuries is one of the many areas where homeopathic medicine comes into its own. Use of Arnica in an injury not only helps deal with the initial shock but also limits bruising by promoting the reabsorption of blood while minimizing pain. Symphytum promotes the knitting of bones in a fracture and eases pain, while Calendula acts as a natural antiseptic, slowing down bleeding and aiding the healing of tissue. In all these situations, the homeopathic medicines are acting as catalysts, speeding up the processes that would naturally happen in the body given time. The advantages of judicious homeopathic prescribing are obvious in a situation where time is acknowledged as the best healer.

How to Select the Appropriate Homeopathic Medicine

You will find homeopathic prescribing for accidents and injuries a little different from the prescribing outlined in other sections of this book. This is because, for many conditions in this section, initial prescribing is much more routine than in other conditions such as indigestion or coughs and colds. For instance, you will quickly notice that Arnica is universally recommended as the first remedy to take internally if there has been any shock or trauma to the system following injury. In other situations where more differentiation is required, as with sprains and strains, follow the advice given below.

1. Turn to the table entitled Sprains and Strains. Let us say that Arnica has helped the acute phase of injury enormously, but you are left with residual pain that is not being resolved by the remedy. Look down the left-hand column entitled Type to identify which category your symptoms fall into. If you are in pain when you begin movement but feel much better once you have gotten going, the chances are that the information given for "Sprains and strains that feel better with continued movement" is for you.
2. Check the General Indications to see if these symp-

toms fit your own. If you have pains associated with muscular overexertion that feel relieved by continued, gentle movement, then it looks as though you are on the right track.

3. Finally, check the Worse From and Better From columns to see if these also fit. Do bear in mind that these two columns do not just refer to what makes your sprain or strain better or worse, but also to what might make you *generally* feel better or worse. So if you have definitely noticed that you feel worse from exposure to damp and cold but taking a warm bath or staying warm in bed helps your pain, the chances are that Rhus tox. is the remedy for you.

For information on how to take the appropriate remedy, see the section entitled How to Take Homeopathic Medicines (p. 8) in the chapter on practical homeopathy; exactly the same principles apply.

Remember that in first-aid situations it is appropriate to take one remedy internally and to use another topically on the skin in gel, cream, or ointment form. For example, if you have sustained a cut after a fall, it is fine to take Arnica internally while you bathe the cut with diluted Calendula tincture. Do bear in mind that Arnica cream or gel should only be applied to bruises where the skin is unbroken; **do not** apply it to cuts or grazes. In the latter situation, Calendula would be the most appropriate choice of gel or ointment.

CUTS AND BRUISES

TYPE	GENERAL INDICATIONS	WORSE FROM	BETTER FROM	REMEDY
Simple cuts and grazes	Cuts that are straightforward with no signs of sepsis.	Chill	Being still	**Calendula** *The remedy may be applied in gel, ointment, or diluted tincture, any of which may be applied directly to the wound.*
Deep cuts with nerve involvement.	Pains are shooting, and there is a general hypersensitivity to touch.	Touch Moving	Being still	**Hypericum** *Very useful for injuries to parts rich in nerves: fingers, toes, and soles of feet.*
Incised wounds	Clean cuts with stinging, lacerated sensations.	Motion Pressure	Heat	**Staphysagria** *Often indicated in injury from sharp instruments.*

CUTS AND BRUISES (cont.)

Type	General Indications	Worse From	Better From	Remedy
Simple bruising, early stages	Sore, aching and bruised sensations that make someone feel very restless and uncomfortable.	Exertion Touch	Resting with head lower than the body	**Arnica** *Also indicated for the general sytemic trauma following a fall or accident. The remedy may be taken internally and applied to the bruised area in cream or ointment form,* provided the skin surface has not been cut.
Black eyes or bruises that feel better when treated with cold applications	(See Remedy)	Heat Moving	Cool air Cold bathing Resting	**Ledum** *May be indicated after Arnica has reached the end of its usefulness. Often helps ease the pain and speed up the healing of bruised tissue around the eye area.*
Bruising as a result of injury to the eyeball or bones around the eye	(See Remedy)	Touch		**Symphytum** *May be indicated after Arnica if swelling has subsided, but pain persists. Often helpful after injury to the eye from a blunt object.*

CUTS AND BRUISES (cont.)

Type	General Indications	Worse From	Better From	Remedy
Bruises of the shin bone, kneecap, or elbow	Area is generally sore, bruised, and lame.	Lying Sitting Going up or down stairs	Warmth Rubbing	**Ruta** *Very strongly indicated for bruises involving the periosteum (the membranous sheath that provides a covering for bones).*
Very deep bruising to tissues	(See Remedy)	Touch Hot bath	Moving Cold applied locally	**Bellis perennis** *May be indicated after a heavy blow that results in bruising of deep tissue, e.g., a blow to the breasts. May also be of use after bruising of deeper tissues following surgery.*

The following will be helpful in addition to selecting the appropriate homeopathic remedy;

1. Where the skin has been broken, be sure to bathe the wound, removing any visible dirt. Examine the wound thoroughly before applying a sterile dressing, to make sure no dirt has been left embedded in the skin.
2. When bathing a cut, Calendula tincture **diluted** in boiled, cooled water makes an excellent antiseptic solution. Calendula will help speed up healing of lacerated tissue, aid in stopping bleeding, and act as a natural antiseptic inhibiting infection. When diluting the tincture use 1 part tincture to 10 parts boiled, cooled water.
3. Calendula gel or ointment also makes an excellent antiseptic agent when applied to clean skin after bathing with diluted Calendula tincture. For grazed wounds, calendula ointment is more appropriate.
4. Bear in mind that a wide cut may need stitches. If not, bringing the edges of the wound together and covering the area with a sterile gauze bandage may be sufficient.
5. If bruising has occurred and the skin has not been broken, applying ice packs to the injured area for twenty or thirty minutes will help reduce swelling.
6. For bruised tissue where the skin has not been broken, Arnica cream or ointment may be applied directly to the skin. This will act in tandem with internal administration of the remedy, relieving pain and speeding up the healing process.

If any of the following occur, seek professional help:

1. Any bleeding that is profuse or associated with any numbness or tingling of the injured part, or general loss of strength.
2. Deep cuts sustained to the chest, face, or abdomen.
3. Deep, wide cuts that refuse to be held together with adhesive bandages; in cases like these, stitches are likely to be required.
4. Dirt is very deeply embedded and cannot be expelled by bathing and cleaning.
5. Any sign of infection around a wound, especially affecting the palm of the hand or the undersides of the fingers.
6. Someone shows signs of repeated, easy bruising.

PUNCTURE WOUNDS

Type	General Indications	Worse From	Better From	Remedy
Puncture wounds that feel better when treated with cold applications	Redness and swelling with throbbing pains. The wound feels cold to the touch and feels better when the affected area is bathed with cold water. Stinging and pricking pains.	Warmth	Cold bathing	**Ledum** *The first remedy to consider in puncture wounds.*
Puncture wounds with lots of pink, swollen skin	Lots of sensations of heat and stinging pains that feel much worse when warmth is applied. The site of the wound is extremely swollen and puffy.	Heat Touch	Cool air Cold bathing	**Apis**
Puncture wounds with sharp, shooting pains	Intolerable shooting pains with lacerating sensations. Pains shoot from the site of injury along the affected limb. Wound feels extremely sensitive to touch.	Touch Jarring		**Hypericum**

The following measures will be helpful in addition to selecting the appropriate homeopathic remedy:

1. Try to clean the wound as thoroughly as you can, letting it bleed for a while to remove foreign bodies, germs, and debris. If bleeding is severe, apply pressure to the appropriate point above the artery (see a first-aid manual for specific instructions), but do not exert pressure over the wound itself. This helps avoid pushing any foreign bodies deeper into the wound.
2. Soaking the wounded area is helpful since it has the dual advantage of keeping the wound open to expel any foreign bodies and germs, and of bringing blood to the area, which will speed the healing process. This may be done up to four times a day for about twenty minutes for as long as the pain continues.
3. Applying diluted Hypericum tincture (1 part tincture to 10 parts water) to the wound will greatly ease the pain and speed up healing while the appropriate homeopathic remedy is being taken internally.

If any of the following occur, seek professional help:

1. Puncture wounds that remain tender in excess of two days.
2. Puncture wounds affecting the hands rather than the fingers.
3. Any sign of infection around a puncture wound.
4. Deep puncture wounds or those that are located anywhere except the extremities.
5. Joints affected by puncture wounds, especially if you observe any signs of infection.
6. Any indications of the onset of tetanus (symptoms include rigidity of injured limb, and painful spasms of spinal and abdominal muscles).

STRAINS AND SPRAINS

Type	General Indications	Worse From	Better From	Remedy
Early stage with much swelling and bruised pain	Lots of swelling around the affected area with signs of inflammation and bruising. Soreness and aching that is aggravated by movement.	Moving Touch		**Arnica** *Also useful for general shock associated with injury. May be useful for general strain associated with overexertion.*
Strains and sprains that are made much worse by the slightest movement	Lots of inflammation with rosy red swelling, but not as extreme as sprains and strains requiring Arnica. Generally much better if kept still and made very much worse by any movement. Sharp, stitching pains.	Any slight movement Continued motion	Rest Pressure	**Bryonia**
Strains and sprains that feel better with continued movement	Symptoms are often connected to muscular overexertion. Pain may occur once movement has begun, but will begin to be relieved once movement is under way. Symptoms generally worsen at night.	Initial motion Exposure to cold	Continued motion Warmth	**Rhus tox.** *Often needed, like Bryonia, once the most acute stage of injury has passed.*

STRAINS AND SPRAINS (cont.)

Type	General Indications	Worse From	Better From	Remedy
Torn ligaments and tendons; later stages	Pains may feel bruised and aching and may have been helped initially by Arnica and Rhus tox. May respond badly to cold.	Cold Resting Walking out-of-doors	Warmth Moving indoors	**Ruta** *Particularly for ankle and wrist joints. Especially useful for frozen shoulder and tennis elbow.*
Sprained ankles that feel better when treated with cold	Injured part may feel cold to the touch, and the pain may be relieved by cold applications or cold bathing. Lots of stiffness with pain. Symptoms generally worsen at night.	Heat Walking	Cool bathing Resting	**Ledum**

Apart from selecting the appropriate homeopathic remedy, the following measures will be helpful in speeding up the healing process:

1. Apply ice packs to the injured area (provided the skin is not broken) and elevate the affected limb.
2. Warm applications may be soothing after the first twenty-four to forty-eight hours. Hot or warm bathing may also be soothing.
3. Rest the injured part as much as possible, since overuse of an injured tendon or ligament may cause further damage.
4. If injury to the joint is mild, gentle massage may be very soothing.
5. Do not be tempted to start overusing the joint before it has fully healed. Tendons and ligaments may take six weeks or more to heal.

If any of the following occur, seek professional help:

1. The joint cannot be straightened.
2. Any visible signs of distortion or looseness of the joint.
3. Marked swelling or pain that does not subside after self-help measures have been administered.
4. Any signs of the limb looking blue beyond the injury, or feeling cold or numb.
5. A joint cannot bear weight or be used for between twelve to twenty-four hours after the injury has occurred.

In addition, take special care with children who fall on an outstretched hand and injure the wrist. Fractures of the bones of the wrist often occur this way and special care may be needed in picking these children up.

FRACTURES

Type*	General Indications	Worse From	Better From	Remedy
Fracture that has just occurred	Systemic shock, trauma, and local tenderness. The person may feel dazed after the injury, and there is likely to be a lot of localized bruising and swelling.	Being touched	Lying with head low	**Arnica**
Fractures associated with severe pain but little swelling	Pains are violent and aching and may be associated with feelings of systemic weakness.	Pressure to injured part Cold	Speaking to the injured person	**Eupatorium perfoliatum**
Fractured ribs that feel much worse from the slightest movement	Because of the sensitivity to movement, the injured person feels they must keep very still. Longs to take a deep breath in, but can't because of the pain. May get relief from lying on the injured side.	Moving Heat	Lying motionless Firm pressure	**Bryonia**

*Also indicates stage or progression of fracture

FRACTURES (cont.)

TYPE	GENERAL INDICATIONS	WORSE FROM	BETTER FROM	REMEDY
Fractures that have been set in place	See remedy	Touch		**Symphytum** *Useful for the stage when the initial swelling and pain have subsided, and the knitting of the bone needs to be speeded up. Since this remedy is very efficient at promoting the speedy knitting of bone, always make sure the bones have been set in alignment before administering it.*
Fractures that refuse to knit speedily, even after the use of Symphytum	Slow-knitting bones with sensations of numbness and stiffness as well as pain.	Changes of weather Cold	Warm, dry weather	**Calcarea phos.**

In addition to selecting the appropriate homeopathic medicine, the following measures will be helpful:

1. If you suspect an injury may involve a fracture, keep the limb as still as possible and seek professional help.
2. If the skin has not been broken, ice packs will be useful as a way of keeping swelling down.

If any of the following occur, professional help is indicated:

1. The person who has sustained the injury seems faint, sweaty or pale.
2. You suspect a serious injury of the neck or back, or the person is unconscious.
3. Any signs of distortion to the injured area.
4. Indications of blueness, coldness, or numbness associated with the limb beyond the injured area.
5. Any possible fracture to the thigh or pelvis.
6. Signs of severe bruising or bleeding under the skin around the injured area,
7. The limb is unusable within twelve hours after the injury.

BURNS

Type	General Indications	Worse From	Better From	Remedy
First-degree burns	Stinging pains wtih intense burning.	Touch		**Urtica urens** *May be used internally, or as a diluted tincture directly on skin. Also consider Calendula tincture.*
Second-degree burns	Stinging pains with intense burning.			**Hypericum tincture** *diluted and* **urtica urens** *Taken internally. Once blisters have broken, switch to diluted Calendula tincture.*
Third-degree burns (1)	Cutting, burning, and smarting pains; skin feels raw. Pain and inflammation is violently acute. Acute blistering.	Warmth	Cold applied locally	**Cantharis** *Taken internally.*

BURNS (cont.)

Type	General Indications	Worse From	Better From	Remedy
Third-degree burns (2)	Tearing, drawing, burning pains leading to trembling.	Drafts	Avoiding extremes of heat or cold	**Causticum** *Indicated for the effects of deep burns. May also be helpful in resolving old burns that are still painful.*
Electrical burns				**Phosphorus**

In addition to giving the appropriate homeopathic remedy, it is worthwhile bearing the following in mind:

1. First and straightforward second-degree burns may be treated at home. Third-degree burns and more serious second-degree burns will need attention in an emergency room as soon as possible.
2. Avoid breaking blisters, as this may cause wound to become infected. If a blister breaks spontaneously, use Calendula gel or ointment, or diluted Calendula tincture to inhibit infection. Dressings should be changed two or three times a day.
3. For straightforward first-degree burns, apply cold water to the burn until the pain has eased. Then apply the appropriate diluted tincture as well as taking the indicated remedy internally.
4. Do not try to remove any clothing from a third-degree burn. While waiting for help, try to reassure the person as much as possible.

If any of the following occur, seek professional help:

1. Any third-degree burn. Watch for symptoms of shock; these are:
   - Confusion or unconsciousness
   - Weakness
   - Irregular or shallow breathing
   - Coldness and pale skin
2. Any sign of infection involving swelling, redness, or pus around the area of the burn.

SHOCK

TYPE	GENERAL INDICATIONS	WORSE FROM	BETTER FROM	REMEDY
Shock associated with physical trauma	(See Remedy)	Being approached Touched	Lying with head low	**Arnica** *Most often indicated after a fall or accident involving lots of bruising. Swelling, bruised pain, and possible injuries to the head and neck would suggest the appropriateness of this remedy*
Shock symptons with marked need for fresh air	State of collapse; skin has a blue tinge and feels cold and clammy to the touch. A strong desire may be expressed for being fanned, which alleviates the general condition.	Warmth Pressure of clothes	Being fanned Cool air Elevating feet	**Carbo veg.**
Shock with severe anxiety and restlessness	Shock may follow a life-threatening situation, where the person may be left with a conviction that they are about to die. Breathing is rapid, and palpitations occur with a heightened anxiety state. Sweating may occur with marked trembling.	Chill Noise Light	Rest Open air	**Aconitum**

Get professional help as quickly as possible. While waiting for help, the following measures will be helpful in addition to giving the appropriate homeopathic remedy:

1. Reassure the patient as much as possible.
2. Loosen clothing at the neck, waist, and chest.
3. Try to avoid exposing the patient to extremes of heat and cold.
4. On no account move the patient if you suspect a serious injury.
5. Patient's legs may be elevated slightly higher than the chest.

SUNSTROKE/HEAT PROSTRATION

Type	General Indications	Worse From	Better From	Remedy
Sunstroke with throbbing headache that is relieved by bending the head backward	Bright red, dry skin that radiates heat. Hot sensations may alternate with chills, and there may be an absence of thirst with fever. Throbbing sensations with headache are likely to be aggravated by lying down in a darkened room. Pains move in a downward direction.	Noise Light Jarring Lying flat	Bending head back Sitting propped up in bed in a darkened room— *not* lying flat which aggravates	**Belladonna**
Sunstroke with throbbing headaches made worse by bending head back	Similar to sunstroke treated with Belladonna, but with less burning of the skin. Headache responds well to cool, open air. Ice packs to the head make it feel worse. Head pain accelerates with sunrise and decreases in intensity with sunset. Pains move in an upward direction.	Bending head back Cold applications	Cool, fresh air Being uncovered Pressure	**Glonoinum**
Heat exhaustion with cramps	Rapid pulse with nausea, faintness, coldness, and pallor. Cramps occur with jerking of muscles ending in possible convulsions. Picture of great weakness and collapse, with clammy, profuse sweats.	Touch Motion Raising arms	Cold drinks	**Cuprum**

Type	General Indications	Worse From	Better From	Remedy
Heat exhaustion with extreme coldness of body and general stiffness	Faintness and heat stroke with rapid pulse and nausea. Sweating is extremely profuse and clammy and accompanied by pallor. Face may be tinged with blue.	Touch	Covering Lying down	**Veratrum album**

The following advice will be helpful in addition to selecting the appropriate homeopathic remedy:

1. Cool the person down as quickly as possible by removing clothing and keeping them in a cool environment. Fanning and cool bathing will also help the cooling process.
2. If the temperature is not dangerously raised, sipping from a large glass of water in which a half a teaspoonful of salt has been dissolved will help guard against muscle cramps and dehydration.
3. If there are any signs of drowsiness, unconsciousness, severe headache, rapid pulse, nausea, convulsions, or vomiting, send for help as quickly as possible. If patient is unconscious, treat for shock (see p. 33) while you are waiting for help to arrive.
4. If the temperature is dangerously high (103 or above) get help as quickly as possible while you attempt to get the temperature down. **Do bear in mind that sunstroke is potentially a very serious condition that requires prompt emergency treatment: If in doubt, get medical help immediately.**

INSECT BITES AND STINGS

Type	General Indications	Worse From	Better From	Remedy
Bites or stings with marked swelling and puffiness	Much localized redness, stinging, pain, heat, and swelling. Reacts well to cool applications, while pain is made worse by heat.	Heat Touch	Cool bathing Cool applications	**Apis** *Very useful in cases of urticaria that develop after a sting.*
Bites and stings that feel cold, but are relieved by cold applications	Stinging and pricking pains that are relieved by cool bathing. The area affected by the bite or sting may feel cold to the touch. Lots of swelling and redness accompany discomfort.	Warmth	Cold bathing	**Ledum**
Urticaria that develops after a sting	Stinging and burning pains with raised red blotches. Itching is maddeningly intense.	Cool bathing Touch	Heat	**Urtica urens**

INSECT BITES AND STINGS (cont.)

Type	General Indications	Worse From	Better From	Remedy
Large and irritating mosquito bites	Stinging, smarting pains accompany mosquito bites. Extreme sensitivity to discomfort.	Touch	Warmth Rest	**Staphysagria**

If someone is suffering from the effects of a sting, in addition to taking the appropriate homeopathic remedy, try to remove any sting remaining in the wound and apply cold compresses.

If any of the following occur, seek professional help:

1. Any symptoms of rapidly advancing swelling, especially affecting the mouth and throat.
2. Signs of breathing problems.
3. Confusion, fainting, or loss of consciousness.
4. You have any knowledge that the person affected has a history of allergy to insect or bee/wasp stings.

DENTAL WORK PROBLEMS

TYPE	GENERAL INDICATIONS	WORSE FROM	BETTER FROM	REMEDY
Bruised pain following any dental work except wisdom tooth extractions	Trauma and bruising to tissue in the mouth caused by any type of dental work.	Any slight touch		**Arnica** *Excellent as a first choice of remedy. Avoid giving Arnica after extraction of wisdom teeth, since it is so effective at promoting reabsorption of blood, it can lead to a dry socket. In the event of an extraction, choose an alternative appropriate remedy.*
Nerve pains following drilling or extraction	Shooting, violent pains that seem to radiate from the point of injury.			**Hypericum** *Often needed if there is discomfort following injection of anesthetic*
Pains relating to site of injection	Discomfort at the area where injection has been given. Painful area may feel cold, but the pain feels better when treated with cold applications.	Heat applied to painful area	Cold bathing of injured area	**Ledum**

DENTAL WORK PROBLEMS (cont.)

TYPE	GENERAL INDICATIONS	WORSE FROM	BETTER FROM	REMEDY
Deep aching that has not been resolved by using Arnica	Deep aching pains that convey the feeling that bones have been bruised.	Cold	Warmth	**Ruta** *Often helpful in cases of dry socket. Not likely to be indicated in the early stages following dental work.*
Excessive bleeding following tooth extractions	Profuse bleeding even from a small wound. Possible anxiety with bleeding and need for reassurance.			**Phosphorus**
Pains after a filling or extraction, with physical and mental hypersensitivity.	Terrific irritability with pain; can't stand exposure to cold in any form. Pain relieved by warm applications. May be snappy and just want to be left alone to go to sleep.	Cold Noise Touch	Napping Keeping warm	**Nux vomica**

DENTAL WORK PROBLEMS (cont.)

TYPE	GENERAL INDICATIONS	WORSE FROM	BETTER FROM	REMEDY
Severe sharp pains following dental work	Pains are stabbing and very severe. Wound feels lacerated with stinging, smarting pains. Feelings of resentment following dental work.	Touch Cold drinks	Warmth Rest	**Staphysagria**
Pre–dental work "nerves"	Terrific feeling of anxiety and fear with awful restlessness. May feel so bad that death seems preferable to state of nervous tension. Mounting feeling of terror as appointment approaches.			**Aconitum**

In addition to selecting the appropriate homeopathic remedy, the following suggestions may be helpful:

1. Use a mouthwash of Calendula or Hypericum tincture. Dilute 40 drops of tincture in 1/4 pint of boiled, cooled water and rinse around your mouth at regular intervals for a couple of days. This will inhibit infection and speed up healing.
2. If you find a visit to the dentist very traumatic, try to have an afternoon appointment so that you can go home and rest afterward in order to give your body a chance to recover. Above all, don't force yourself to do something strenuous or demanding if you don't feel up to it.
3. If you have any doubts about the time it is taking your mouth to heal, or if pain seems to be continuing for longer than you would expect, do consult your dentist for advice.

BLEEDING

TYPE	GENERAL INDICATIONS	WORSE FROM	BETTER FROM	REMEDY
Bleeding following injury	Bleeding associated with shock or after sustaining an injury.	Any slight touch	Lying down	**Arnica** *This is one of the first remedies to consider in any trauma state.*
Bleeding associated with fainting	Bleeding is accompanied by blue-tinged pallor, clammy sweat, and air hunger. The nature of the bleeding is steady and oozing.	Warm rooms	Fanning with cool air	**Carbo veg.**
Bleeding with nauseous sensations and possible shortness of breath	Bleeding is bright red and comes in spurts or gushes. Symptoms may be accompanied by feeble pulse and cold sweat. Nausea is made much worse by movement.	Warmth Lying down	Open air Rest	**Ipecac**

BLEEDING (cont.)

TYPE	GENERAL INDICATIONS	WORSE FROM	BETTER FROM	REMEDY
Recurrent nosebleeds or small wounds that bleed profusely	Recurrent nosebleeds are often sparked off by overvigorous nose blowing.	Touch Any exertion	Open air Cold water Sleep	**Phosphorus** *Should be considered for any minor wound that bleeds excessively.*

In addition to giving the appropriate homeopathic medicine, try to ensure that bleeding is either stopping or under control; the following measures will also be helpful:

1. Try direct pressure over the wound (provided it is not a puncture wound where something has remained embedded in it). You should see a reduction in the flow of blood in fifteen minutes.
2. Place a sterile dressing over the wound, ensuring that it extends beyond the edges. Secure firmly, but not with so much pressure that it interferes with circulation.
3. In nosebleeds, ensure that the patient leans well forward and advise them to breathe through the mouth while pinching the soft part of the nose. Any blood in the mouth should be spat out to avoid vomiting. If nosebleeds are associated with an injury to the head, get professional advice.
4. If you are in any doubt, always get help as quickly as possible.

3

Homeopathy for Sore Throats, Coughs, and Colds

THE RESPIRATORY SYSTEM

Breathing is essential to life, as it is the process by which we take in oxygen, which is used up by the body, and eliminate the byproduct carbon dioxide. Following the path of the air, respiration starts at the nose or mouth where air is breathed in and down the windpipe into the lungs. In the lungs, oxygen is absorbed into the bloodstream to be pumped around the body by the heart. Meanwhile carbon dioxide and water vapor, which can't be used by the body, are released by the blood into the lungs to be breathed out.

Without the exchange of carbon dioxide and oxygen involved in the process of breathing, life could not be maintained. Seen from this viewpoint, optimum functioning of the respiratory system (the organs and blood involved in the process) is vital to maintaining good health. Short-lived disorders such as the common cold can cause a great deal of discomfort by disrupting the smooth functioning of the respiratory system, and the search for an orthodox medical cure still continues.

Basic drugs used in treating sore throats, coughs, and hay fever include antibiotics, cough suppressants or expectorants, and antihistamines. Prophylactic measures are now also adopted such as the administration of a flu immunization before the winter season begins in the hope that it will reduce the number of colds suffered by the patient. The main thrust of the orthodox approach is involved with reducing inflammatory processes that result in fever, mucous production, and general irritation of mucous membranes.

Homeopathic Medicines and the Respiratory System

The homeopathic approach views cold and cough symptoms as the body's mechanism of ridding itself of noxious material. In this light, one can see how mucous discharges are a basic mechanism in flushing toxins out of the body. The coughing reflex can also be seen to be fulfilling the same function as it attempts to expel the byproducts of acute infection. When these processes go on too long, they are unable to carry out their task and result in making the person more and more exhausted and unwell. Instead of attempting to suppress these symptoms, homeopathic medicines work by giving them a boost and enabling them to carry on the job efficiently and quickly.

For this reason, after an appropriate homeopathic medicine has been administered, the symptoms occasionally appear to be intensified for a short while as the body rids itself of toxic waste. If this is the result of the homeopathic medicine, although the symptoms are still present, there will be a general improvement in the sense of well-being and vitality. In other words, although the person still has their sore throat or cold, they feel much better in themselves, which is a sign that improvement of the specific symptoms should rapidly follow.

How to Select the Appropriate Homeopathic Medicine

If you have turned to this section of the book because you have just developed the first signs of a cold, this is how to select your homeopathic remedy:

1. Turn to the table entitled Colds and look down the left-hand column entitled Type to identify which category your symptoms fall into. If, for example you have recently been exposed to a chill and started to feel ill soon afterward, the chances are that the information given for "Early stage, after exposure to dry, cold winds" is likely to be most useful.

2. Check the General Indications in the next column to see if these symptoms fit your own. If you have lots of sneezing, feel thirsty, and have generally seemed anxious and restless since the symptoms developed, it looks like you are still on the right track. If, on the other hand, you have a high temperature, look flushed, and generally feel feverish and irritable, take a look at the entries for colds treated with other early onset remedies, such as Belladonna and Ferrum phos. Remember that you are looking for the general symptom picture that most closely matches your own.

3. Finally check the Worse From and Better From columns to see if these also fit. Do bear in mind that these two columns do not just refer to what makes your cold symptoms better or worse, but also what might make you generally feel better or worse. So if, for example, you have definitely noticed that you feel much worse at night, or when in a warm room, but fresh air makes you feel better, the chances are that Aconite will be the best remedy for you.

4. Remember that a cold generally passes through a

number of different stages before it resolves itself, and that you are likely to need a change of remedy at each stage. In other words, once you have passed the stage of initial onset, Aconitum is no longer likely to be appropriate to your symptoms. Just take note of any changes; e.g., if you begin to develop a cough, use the same method described above to find what the most appropriate remedy is likely to be. You may also combine tables (e.g., if you have both a sore throat and cough at the same time), always remembering that you are looking for the single homeopathic remedy that covers the whole symptom picture most adequately.

5. It is unlikely that taking a homeopathic remedy will abort a cold, but if the selection of remedy is appropriate, it will take you through the various stages quickly, and with the minimum amount of discomfort.

For information on how to take the appropriate remedy, see the section entitled How to Take Homeopathic Medicines (p. 8) in the chapter on practical homeopathy; exactly the same principles apply.

SORE THROATS/TONSILITIS: EARLY STAGE

Type	General Indications	Worse From	Better From	Remedy
Sore throat with high fever	Very bright red throat with lots of pain when trying to swallow liquids. Aversion to drinking. "Strawberry" tongue (covered with bright red spots). Dry mouth and throat. Pains may extend to right ear on swallowing. Generally red, flushed, and feverish.	Drinking Talking Empty swallowing	Rest in bed	**Belladonna** *Most useful in the first 24 hours.*
Sore throat with fear and anxiety	Sore throat may come on after exposure to cold or drafts. Fever may be high with fear and restlessness. Inflammation of throat with pains. Desire to swallow that aggravates feeling of constriction and pain. Symptoms generally worsen at night.	Extreme changes from heat or cold	Open air Sleep	**Aconitum** *Most useful in first 24 hours.*
Sore throats with extreme swelling	Glossy, "water-bag" appearance (as though filled with water) to the throat, tonsils, and tongue. Pains are characteristically stinging and hot.	Warm drinks Touch	Cold drinks Cool surroundings	**Apis**

SORE THROATS/TONSILITIS: ESTABLISHED STAGE

Type	General Indications	Worse From	Better From	Remedy
Left-sided pain with lots of constriction	Pain often starts on the left side and extends to the ear. Difficulty swallowing because of a sensation of a lump in the throat. Possible ulceration of the throat. Patient dislikes having anything constricting around the neck.	After sleep Empty swallowing Warm drinks Warm rooms	Swallowing food Cold drinks Open air	**Lachesis**
Sore throat with painful, inflamed glands	Ulcerated throat with offensive breath and lots of saliva in the mouth. Pains may begin on the right side and move to the left. Very restless and aggravated by temperature extremes. May be very sweaty.	Night-time Heat of the bed Cold surroundings	Regular temperature	**Mercurius**
Sore throat with aching pains in the body	Generally feels unwell and feverish. Lots of glandular unease and shooting pains to the ears on swallowing. Severe inflammation of the throat that looks very dark red or purple in color. Very chilly, even when covered. Pain at base of tongue when extended.	Hot drinks Right side Cold	Warmth	**Phytolacca**

SORE THROATS/TONSILITIS: ESTABLISHED STAGE

TYPE	GENERAL INDICATIONS	WORSE FROM	BETTER FROM	REMEDY
Sore throat with sharp, splinterlike pains	Very toxic conditions with tendency to pus formation. Ulceration of the throat with a sensation as though there were a fish bone or splinter embedded in it. Shooting pains extending to the ears when not swallowing. Irritability and hypersensitivity with illness. Strong dislike of being cold.	Cold in any form	Warmth	**Hepar sulph.**
Sore throat that begins on the right and moves to the left	Generally slow onset of feeling unwell or malaise. Sensation of lump rising in the throat with constant desire to swallow. Symptoms in general may be aggravated mid-afternoon until early evening. Symptoms worsen at night.	Cold drinks Heat of room	Warm drinks Open air	**Lycopodium**

LARYNGITIS

TYPE	GENERAL INDICATIONS	WORSE FROM	BETTER FROM	REMEDY
Sudden loss of voice from exposure to dry, cold winds	Loss of voice with fever, anxiety, and restlessness. May accompany croupy cough in children. Symptoms generally worsen at night.	Exposure to cold air	Sleep	**Aconitum**
Dry, sore throat with loss of voice	Hoarseness or complete loss of voice with constant desire to clear the throat. Much worse on attempting to speak. Throat feels very dry and sensitive to touch or cold air. Dry tickling cough may accompany loss of voice. Symptoms worsen during evening hours.	Talking Cold air	Sound sleep Reassurance Cool drinks	**Phosphorus**
Loss of voice from emotional upset or shock	Sensation of lump in the throat with constriction. May feel throat is constantly sore since grief or shock.	Dry swallowing Fluids	Swallowing food Distraction	**Ignatia**

Once you have selected the most appropriate homeopathic remedy, the following suggestions may be useful as supportive measures in order to speed up the natural healing process:

1. Take plenty of fluids to keep the temperature down and flush toxins out of the body. Mineral water tends to be best suited to this purpose, rather than warm drinks like coffee or tea, which encourage dehydration.
2. Vitamin C may be useful as a supplement to assist the immune system in fighting the infection. Between 1–3 grams may be taken in a twenty-four-hour period for one to three days. Always reduce the amount of vitamin C taken if diarrhea occurs, since this is a sign that a lower dose is needed. Once the reduction has been made, digestion should return to normal.
3. Avoid foods which are painful to swallow and difficult to digest. Homemade soups and steamed vegetables, fruit, or salads are likely to be most digestible, nutritious, and easy on the throat.
4. Try to rest as much as possible to aid the body in fighting infection.
5. Avoid moving from one extreme of temperature to another, and try to humidify the air by placing containers of water at strategic places, e.g., near radiators.
6. Gargle with a solution of warm water and salt or lemon and honey. A very soothing gargle may also be made by diluting Calendula tincture in warm water.

If any of the following occur, seek professional help:

1. Throat pain is severe with difficulty swallowing.
2. Sore throats in children with fever that looks persistent.
3. A sore throat in anyone who has suffered from rheumatic fever.
4. Sore throats accompanied by a rash and high temperature.
5. Ulceration or pus formation in the throat.
6. Any problems with breathing or drooling accompanying a sore throat.

COLDS

Type*	General Indications	Worse From	Better From	Remedy
Early stage of cold with high temperature	Very hot and feverish with dry, bright red skin. Symptoms come on rapidly and progress quickly. Restlessness and irritability. Pulse may be rapid.	Light Noise Motion	Sitting upright in bed	**Belladonna**
Early stage of cold after exposure to dry, cold winds	Restlessness with strong anxiety. Lots of sneezing with dry sensations in the nose or fluent nasal discharge in the mornings. Throats and chest feel sore and constricted. Thirsty for large quantities of water. Colds may develop after fright or shock. Symptoms worse at night.	Warm room Talking	Open air	**Aconitum**
Early stage of cold with shivering, chills, and feverish symptoms	Not so intensely hot as patients needing Belladonna, or as anxious as those who require Aconitum. Hot face with well-defined circular patches on cheeks. May feel generally heavy and weary. Symptoms generally worsen at night.	Cold air	Warmth Cold applications	**Ferrum phos.**

*Also indicates stage or progression of cold.

COLDS (cont.)

Type	General Indications	Worse From	Better From	Remedy
Cold with lots of sneezing and streaming	Streaming eyes and nose accompany sneezing. Discharges are burning, profuse, and watery. Red, burning, and inflamed eyes with bland discharge. Nasal discharge burns top lip. Symptoms worsen during evening hours.	Warm rooms Indoors	Out-of-doors Cool rooms	**Allium cepa**
Cold with profuse nasal discharge and tears	Fluent, bland nasal discharge with copious burning tears. (The complete opposite of Allium cepa.) Chilliness with frequent sneezing and light sensitivity. Symptoms worsen at night, get better during the day.	Lying down Open air Light		**Euphrasia**
Cold with extreme physical and mental irritability and sensitivity	Slow onset of cold after exposure to dry, cold weather. Lots of sneezing and tickling in the nose, with itching in the ears. Nose runs in warm room and during the day, but feels stuffed up at night. Lots of irritability and physical sensitivity to drafts of colds air.	Eating On waking Cold air Mental exertion Lack of sleep	Warmth Napping	**Nux vomica**

COLDS (cont.)

Type	General Indications	Worse From	Better From	Remedy
Cold with cold sores and dry lips	Lots of nasal discharge that looks like raw egg white. Loss of smell and taste with post-nasal drip. Lips may be cracked in the center. May be depressed with cold symptoms, but aggravated by sympathy and attention.	Sympathy Sunlight Warmth	Open air Not eating	**Natrum mur.**

For general advice on adjunctive ways of dealing with cold symptoms see the following Influenza section.

INFLUENZA

Type	General Indications	Worse From	Better From	Remedy
Rapid onset of symptoms with high temperature	Rapid pulse with very bright red, dry, hot skin. Throbbing pains that are made worse by any movement.	Motion Stimulation Light Noise	Lying semi-upright in bed	**Belladonna** *This remedy is likely to be of most use within the first 24 hours of symptoms developing.*
Flu symptoms with exhaustion and anxiety	Extreme restlessness and anxiety over symptoms. Lots of burning pains that are better when treated with heat (except headache, which may respond better to fresh air). Chilliness with a desire for warmth. Good response to company and distraction.	Night Food Cold	Warmth Company Rest Open air	**Arsenicum album**
Classic flu symptoms with shivering, aching, and fatigue	Slow onset with chills running up and down spine. Heaviness and lethargy with general aches and pains. Possible temperature without thirst. Withdrawn and apathetic.	Change of climate Motion	Urination Alcohol Open air	**Gelsemium**

INFLUENZA (cont.)

Type	General Indications	Worse From	Better From	Remedy
Flu with extreme weakness and aching deep in the bones	Deep aching pains in the back and limbs, bones feel as if they were broken. Desire to keep still because of the degree of pain. Chill and fever with bursting headache. Eyes may feel particularly aching and sore. Bilious feelings with flu.	Cold air Moving	Distraction Warmth	**Eupatorium perfoliatum**
Flu with stiff and aching muscles, much worse at night	May come on after exposure to damp cold weather. Glands are swollen, hard, and painful. Cannot find any position in bed at night that affords any relief. Nose may be congested with thick green mucus. Chilly feelings alternate with flushes of heat. Symptoms worsen at night.	Cold air Rest	Warmth Gentle movement	**Rhus tox.**
Established stage of flu with residual catarrhal symptoms	Changeability of symptoms. Weepiness and feelings of depression with illness, which are improved by consolation and attention. Mucous discharges are bland, thick, and greeny-yellow. Possible discomfort in sinuses and glands. Chilly, but feels better from fresh air.	Stuffy rooms Rest Eating	Cool air Gentle motion Crying	**Pulsatilla**

The following measures may be helpful in addition to selecting the appropriate homeopathic remedy:

1. Stay in as constant a temperature as possible, especially if you suspect your temperature may be high. Moving from one extreme to another is only likely to make you feel worse.

2. It is very important to rest as much as possible to allow the body as much chance as possible to fight the infection. This takes energy, so it is a very good idea not to make any extra demands on your body to allow the natural healing process to take place.

3. Useful supplements include vitamin C and garlic tablets, which are both thought to aid in mobilizing the body's own defenses in dealing with infection. Try 1–3 grams of vitamin C daily for two or three days depending on bowel tolerance, reducing the dosage until the digestion settles down. Two garlic tablets may be taken three times a day for as long as the infection continues.

4. Keep your diet as light as possible and drink as much water as you can to help your body flush out toxins and loosen mucus. Drinking fluids regularly becomes a strong priority if you have a raised temperature.

If any of the following occur, seek professional help:

1. Raised temperature in a baby or young child.
2. Raised temperature accompanied by stiff neck, lethargy, irritability, and changed breathing.
3. Stubborn raised temperature in otherwise fit adults that does not respond to naturopathic or homeopathic measures.

If in doubt get help. It is always best to err on the cautious side, especially where young children or elderly people are concerned, since illnesses can develop rapidly at both sides of the age spectrum.

COUGHS

TYPE*	GENERAL INDICATIONS	WORSE FROM	BETTER FROM	REMEDY
Early stage of cough after exposure to dry, cold winds	Croupy-sounding cough that is particularly disturbing in the later part of the night. Lots of anxiety and restlessness with coughing bouts. Cough may sound barking and choking.	Exposure to cold Talking Smoke	Warm rooms Lying down	**Aconitum**
Dry cough with wheezing; especially bad at night	Lots of restlessness and anxiety with cough; especially marked at night. Cough is dry and tickling, making the person sit up in bed at night for relief. Cough is aggravated by exposure to cold, and relieved by sips of warm drinks. Burning pains in the chest with wheezing.	Cold Night Exertion	Warmth Lying with head elevated Company	**Arsenicum album**
Dry, irritating cough with desire to press on the chest	Hard, dry cough that is made worse entering a warm room. Possible marked thirst for large quantities of cold water. Headache may accompany the cough. Pains in the chest from coughing are relieved by firm pressure, either by lying on the painful area, or pressing the hand firmly agianst it.	Eating Drinking Warm rooms Taking a deep breath	Pressure Fresh air Lying still	**Bryonia**

*Also indicates stage or progression of cough.

COUGHS (cont.)

TYPE	GENERAL INDICATIONS	WORSE FROM	BETTER FROM	REMEDY
Tickling cough wtih hoarseness that is made much worse by talking	Tickly, burning cough that exhausts, caused by head colds that descend to the chest. Mucus discharges are characteristically yellowy-green or containing streaks of blood. Chest may feel tight and heavy.	Changes of temperature Moving Talking Cold drinks	Company Attention Sleep	**Phosphorus** *May be called for in the early stages of bronchitis*
Cough with gagging and retching	Nature of cough resembles whooping cough. Bouts of coughing follow each in close succession. Coughing bouts end in retching. Coughing characteristically comes as soon as the person lies down.	Lying down Eating and drinking	Keeping chest still Open air	**Drosera**
Dry, shallow cough with extreme sensitivity to cold air	Cough set off by breathing in cold air and relieved by staying in constant temperature. Barking, hacking cough that prevents sleep. Cough aggravated by talking and touching the external throat.	Cold air Changes of temperature Lying down	Warm air	**Rumex crispus**

COUGHS (cont.)

TYPE	GENERAL INDICATIONS	WORSE FROM	BETTER FROM	REMEDY
Cough that is so hard and rasping, it sounds like a saw being drawn through dry wood	Dryness of mucous membranes with severe barking cough. Larynx feels obstructed, burning, and dry. May be awakened from sleep by suffocating sensations accompanying the cough.	Very cold drinks Sleep Dry, cold wind	Eating or drinking a little Warmth	**Spongia**
Established stage of cough with copious yellow-green mucous discharges	Cough may alternate between being dry at night, and loose during the day and on waking. Characteristic dry mouth without thirst, and chilliness with desire for open air may accompany the cough. Generally feels better with gentle motion out-of-doors. May be depressed and weepy with the cough.	Stuffy rooms Keeping still	Sitting up in bed Open air Gentle exercise Sympathy	**Pulsatilla**
Cough with brassy sound and stubborn, tough mucus	Tickling sensation at the base of the throat that precedes cough. Lots of stringy, ropy, tough mucus that may be difficult to dislodge. Mucous deposits may lead to sinus pains at the root of the nose.	Eating Damp cold After sleep	Heat Bringing up mucus	**Kali bichrom.** *Most likely to be of use in the later stages of a head cold that has traveled downward.*

General advice for coughs will be basically the same as advice already given in the sections on colds and flu with the addition of the following:

1. Avoid milk and milk products if you have a cough, since these foods are mucus-forming and can aggravate a cough, especially if taken before bedtime.
2. Try to avoid dry atmospheres by placing containers of water near sources of heat or making use of a commercially manufactured humidifier. If coughing is paricularly troublesome, spending some time in a steam-filled bathroom may help breathing temporarily.

If any of the following occur, seek professional help:

1. Wheezing that occurs in someone who has not experienced this before.
2. Marked chest pain.
3. Accelerated breathing or breathing difficulties, especially in young children.
4. You suspect any foreign body has been inhaled.
5. Any signs of confusion or drowsiness.
6. A cough has persisted with no observable improvement, accompanied by a general decline in energy and well-being.

SINUSITIS

TYPE	GENERAL INDICATIONS	WORSE FROM	BETTER FROM	REMEDY
Sinus pain made worse by touch or exposure to cold	Sensitivity to even the slightest draft of cold air. Also strong irritability and emotional sensitivity. Pain may be concentrated at the base of the nose, and the whole skull may feel bruised.	Cold Touch Dry winds	Heat Moist air	**Hepar sulph.**
Pain and congestion located specifically at the root of the nose	Lots of nasal mucus that is very tough and stringy. General soreness in facial bones, with shooting pains in the sinuses in the region of the cheeks. Pulsating pains and dryness of mucous membranes.	Stooping Damp weather Cold weather Motion	Warmth Pressure	**Kali bichrom.**
Sinus pains improved by wrapping up warmly	Pains often come on after getting wet and chilled. There may be hard crusting in the nose and at the meeting places of mucous membranes and skin. Pains are markedly improved by exertion of pressure to the painful spot.	Cold Noise Motion Talking	Warmth Pressure	**Silica**

SINUSITIS (cont.)

Type	General Indications	Worse From	Better From	Remedy
Sinus pain from long-standing catarrhal conditions with bland, yellow-green mucus	Loss of smell with sinus pains. Nose is stuffed up in the evening and night, but mucus flows more freely in the morning. Nose also feels more stuffed up in warm rooms and feels more comfortable out-of-doors. Weepiness and desire for sympathy may accompany sinus symptoms. Symptoms worsen at night.	Stuffy rooms Heat	Open air Gentle motion Cold in general	**Pulsatilla**
Sinus pains that are raw and burning with offensive nasal discharges	Pressured feeling in bones of the face with sensation of swelling inside the nose. Thin nasal discharges changing to thick offensive mucus. Marked increase in amount of saliva in the mouth, tongue may seem swollen. Generally feels chilly and sweaty. Symptoms worsen at night.	Extreme temperature changes Cold drafts	Moderate temperature Rest	**Merc sol.**

Follow the general suggestions in the preceding sections to help deal with inflamed sinuses.

If any of the following occur, seek professional help:

1. High temperature and/or offensive nasal discharges accompanying sinus pain.
2. Pain is severe and fails to respond to homeopathic treatment in approximately twenty-four hours.

While the following may be useful in giving acute relief during the summer season for hay fever symptoms, it is recommended that long-term homeopathic treatment from a trained practitioner be sought in order to deal with the predisposition to the condition.

HAY FEVER

TYPE	GENERAL INDICATIONS	WORSE FROM	BETTER FROM	REMEDY
Hay fever symptoms with extreme swelling and puffiness	Eyes and throat are exceptionally red and puffy. Swelling looks like water bags and are accompanied by stinging pains. Symptoms are generally strongly aggravated by heat and improved by cold.	Heat Touch Lying down	Cold air and cold bathing	**Apis**
Hay fever accompanied by burning, scanty mucous discharges	Lots of burning accompanying scanty, clear nasal discharge. Better response to warmth than cold. May feel very anxious and restless with symptoms. Eyes are likely to be watery and very sensitive to light, with peripheral swelling. Symptoms worsen at night.	Cold Being outside	Warmth Inside Rest	**Arsenicum album**

HAY FEVER (cont.)

Type	General Indications	Worse From	Better From	Remedy
Hay fever with profuse, clear discharges	Frequent, violent sneezing with accompanying profuse watery discharges from eyes and nose. May develop cold sores after exposure to sunlight, or cracked lips.	Sunlight Warmth Exertion Sympathy	Open air Cool Being left alone	**Natrum mur.**
Hay fever with extreme sensitivity on both physical and emotional levels	Terrific sensitivity to drafts of cold air, light, and odors. Eyes may be blood-shot and watery, and sneezing is likely to be violent and frequent, especially on waking. Very irritable and bad-tempered, which is worse early in the day but gets better as the day goes on.	Odors Stimulation Cold air	Damp weather Warmth In the evening	**Nux vomica**
Hay fever with very bland, thick discharges	Blocked nasal passages feel much worse indoors, especially in a stuffy room. Generally improved by being in the open air. Nose blocks at night, and runs more fluently in the day. May feel chilly, but still desires to be out-of-doors. Symptoms worsen at night.	Warmth Rest	Open air Gentle motion Consolation Cold applications	**Pulsatilla**

Type	General Indications	Worse From	Better From	Remedy
Hay fever with bland discharge from eyes, but acrid discharge from nasal passages	Lots of sneezing with profuse, bland discharge from eyes, which smart. Burning of the upper lip from thin, watery discharge from nose.	Warmth Damp weather	Cool, open air Motion	**Allium cepa**
Hay fever with bland nasal discharge, and acrid tears from eyes	Profuse, hot, acrid tears that require frequent wiping. Eyes are very bloodshot and sensative to light. Lots of bland nasal mucus with possible chest involvement.	Sunlight Wind Warm rooms	Open air Wiping eyes	**Euphrasia**
Hay fever with very persistent sneezing that may be abortive	Intense itching in nose with strong desire to rub it. Tickling sensation in nose may spread over whole body. Extremely sensitive sense of smell with single nostril blocked at one time. Nasal discharge increases even at the thought of the smell of flowers.	Cold air Strong odors Mental exertion	Open air Warmth Eating	**Sabadilla**

The following measures may be helpful in soothing symptoms:

1. Rinse eyes and nasal passages with sterile water.
2. Inhaling steam may help open swollen airways.
3. Increase your fluid intake (preferably water).
4. Avoid substances that are likely to irritate your allergy further, such as dust, perfume, or animal hair.

GENERAL ADVICE

With disorders of the respiratory system such as colds and sore throats, it is worth saying that it is not always necessary to prescribe homeopathic medicines to get over the condition. Very often, the general hints given at the end of each section are enough on their own to make you sufficiently comfortable to get over the illness speedily and well. If, on the other hand, while you are following the general advice, the symptoms are making you feel very unwell, prescribing the appropriate homeopathic medicine at the right time will help enormously in speeding up the healing process and improving your general sense of well-being.

4

Homeopathy for
Digestive Upsets

THE DIGESTIVE SYSTEM

Looked at from a mechanistic standpoint, the digestive system is a food processing machine that opens at one end with the mouth and ends at the other with the anus. In between there are organs that perform certain functions, like the stomach, liver, and intestines, which break down the ingested food into useful or discardable components.

If something goes wrong with this system, the orthodox medical approach involves using drugs to suppress the specific symptom, thus providing a mechanical answer to the problem. In other words, if the problem with the digestive system involves the secretion of too much acid in the stomach, an antacid is used to dilute the stomach secretions temporarily. Or if constipation arises, a laxative is given to stimulate the bowel to evacuate itself more frequently. From these examples it is obvious that orthodox medical drugs work from the premise that when a digestive problem arises, it is that particular compartment of the body that is malfunctioning and requires a mechanical adjustment.

Homeopathic Medicines and the Digestive System

Homeopathic medical theory approaches the concept of disease from a different perspective. Rather than viewing symptoms of illness as an indication that one part of the body alone is in trouble, symptoms are seen as indicators that the whole body has shifted into a state of imbalance. This is particularly relevant to a discussion of digestive problems, since many people experience nausea or acid indigestion as part of an overall systemic response to stress or an overburdened life-style.

The most basic concept in homeopathic theory is that, when well (i.e., in a state of balance), the human body is capable of carrying out all its necessary functions without the help of drugs, because of the presence of biochemical checks and balances that maintain the smooth functioning of the various systems within the body. When stresses occur that knock this self-regulatory functioning off balance, symptoms appear. These are the first indications that all is not well within the body. When the required homeopathic medicine is given at this stage, the body regains its equilibrium and bodily functions are regulated once more to their original smooth functioning.

How to Select the Appropriate Homeopathic Medicine

If you have turned to this section of the book because you are in the throes of a digestive problem like indigestion, this is how you select your homeopathic remedy:

1. Turn to the table entitled Indigestion and look down the left-hand column entitled Type to identify which category your symptoms fall into. If, for example, your stomach normally functions very well but you have had terrible indigestion since you have been given a date for your driving test, the chances are

that the information given for "Indigestion from Anticipation" is for you.

2. Check the General Indications to see if these symptoms fit your own. If you have acid burping and lots of rumbling and gurgling with bloating, then it definitely looks like you are on the right track.

3. Finally check the Worse From and Better From columns to see if these also fit. Do bear in mind that these two columns do not just refer to what makes your indigestion better or worse, but also to what might make you *generally* feel better or worse. So if you have definitely noticed that you feel much worse after eating, but warm drinks or loosening your clothes help your indigestion, the chances are that Lycopodium is the remedy for you.

4. You will find some suggestions at the end of the section on indigestion for general ways of preventing the condition recurring once you have been helped by the indicated remedy.

For information on how to take the appropriate remedy, see the section entitled How to Take Homeopathic Medicines (p. 8) in the chapter on practical homeopathy; exactly the same principles apply.

INDIGESTION

Type	General Indications	Worse From	Better From	Remedy
Indigestion with bloating and excess wind	Extreme swelling around the waist that is much worse after eating anything. Heavy and full sensations in the stomach with violent burping.	Stuffy rooms Tight clothes	Fresh air Passing wind	**Carbo veg.**
Indigeston from anticipation	Bloating with noisy rumbling and gurgling in stomach and abdomen. Eating very little makes the stomach feel full. Acid burping.	Eating a large amount Tight clothes	Warm drinks	**Lycopodium**
Indigestion from fatty, rich foods	Indigestion may follow an overly indigestible meal with lots of red meat or cheese. The mouth may be dry with no thirst, and "repeating" of food eaten hours before. Weepiness may accompany indigestion.	Stuffy rooms Resting	Fresh air Gentle moving Cold drinks	**Pulsatilla**

INDIGESTION (cont.)

Type	General Indications	Worse From	Better From	Remedy
"Morning after" indigestion	A classic hangover headache may accompany the indigestion. Aching may be felt across the eyes or at the back of the head. Sour-tasting burps that are difficult to bring up. Irritability of mind and body.	Any effort Too little sleep	Napping Resting	**Nux vomica**
Acid indigestion from anxiety	Much burning in the stomach relieved by small sips of cold water or tea. Feelings of anxious restlessness with nausea. Prostrated with feelings of sickness. May be chilly with nausea.	Any physical exertion Being chilly	Keeping warm Resting	**Arsenicum album**

Once you have gained relief from a well-chosen homeopathic remedy, the following measures will help prevent the condition occurring again:

1. Eating slowly and trying to relax during a meal are very important ways of preventing indigestion occurring. Eating is a very sensual experience, since more senses than taste alone are brought into play. Lots of people are unaware that digestive juices begin to flow from just smelling and seeing appetizing food, so that the process of digestion can begin long before you put any food into your mouth. Also remember that your stomach is made of muscle, and like any other muscular structure can suffer from tension. If your stomach muscles are in a state of tension when food enters the stomach, the wavelike muscular contractions called *peristalsis* can't happen smoothly. Peristalsis is responsible for smooth digestion, and if it is hampered, the chances are that pain and gas will be the result.

2. Some foods have a bad reputation for contributing to indigestion and are best avoided if you feel an attack developing. The best-known foods in this category are raw onions, peppers, cabbage, and beans. Common irritants of the stomach lining include strong coffee, tea, curries, chilies, and smoking. Very fatty foods like full-fat cheese, cream, and red meat and pork are probably also best avoided if you're feeling queasy.

3. If indigestion or heartburn are persistent and troublesome over a period of time, seek professional help.

VOMITING AND DIARRHEA

TYPE	GENERAL INDICATIONS	WORSE FROM	BETTER FROM	REMEDY
Food Poisoning (1)	Vomiting and diarrhea that occur simultaneously after eating spoiled food. Exhaustion with vomiting to the point of collapse. General sense of chilliness that responds well to warmth. Burning pains relieved by warmth. Restlessness and anxiety with vomiting and diarrhea. Symptoms worsen at night.	Cold Being alone	Resting Warmth (apart from head pain, which is relieved by cold)	**Arsenicum album**
Food Poisoning (2)	Extreme pallor of the face with profuse sweat. Alternating vomiting and diarrhea. Chilly but responds to cool, fresh air. Vomiting is very violent and projectile, preceded by strong feelings of nausea. Overwhelming thirst for cool drinks. Symptoms worsen at night.	Moving Warmth	Rest Cool drinks Lying down	**Veratrum album**
Severe nausea with vomiting	Constant nausea that is not relieved by vomiting. Colicky pains with tender, bloated abdomen. Constant sensation of needing to empty the bowels with nausea. Irritability and oversensitivity.	Extreme cold or heat Moving	Rest Open air	**Ipecac**

VOMITING AND DIARRHEA (cont.)

Type	General Indications	Worse From	Better From	Remedy
Profuse, violent diarrhea	Constant painless diarrhea. Lots of gurgling in bowels. If vomiting occurs with diarrhea the whole abdomen may feel sore. Symptoms worsen in early morning hours.	Hot weather Milk	Rubbing the painful area Lying on the stomach	**Podophyllum**
Upset stomachs from "exam nerves"	"Butterflies" in the stomach with excitement. Loss of appetite with queasy feelings in the stomach. Nervous diarrhea passed without pain. Withdrawal with anxiety.	Anticipation Worry	Relaxation	**Gelsemium**
Diarrhea from fear or excitement	Nausea relieved by eating, which makes the stomach pains worse. Nausea relieved by sour things. Craving for sugar, which aggravates. Noisy belching and severe diarrhea aggravated by eating sweets. Talkativeness and exuberance from "nerves."	Anxiety Closed-in places Sugar	Cool, open air Motion Passing wind	**Argenticum nit.**

In addition to selecting the most helpful homeopathic remedy, the following suggestions may be helpful in cases of vomiting and diarrhea:

1. If vomiting and/or diarrhea occur, the chances are that the digestive tract is attempting to deal with an infection by expelling the contents of the stomach and bowel. In this situation, trying to put more food into the digestive system is counterproductive, so it is best to avoid eating while the vomiting and diarrhea continue. Once things have settled, go back to eating slowly, avoiding any oils, milk, or other fats. The best thing to begin with would be a little brown rice with lightly steamed easily digested vegetables, or a little broth.

2. Although eating is a bad idea during vomiting and diarrhea, drinking is essential to ensure that the body does not get dehydrated. Large quantities of fluid are lost from the body when diarrhea and vomiting occur together, so check the signs listed below if you feel dehydration may be a problem. The best fluid to drink is plain water; avoid milk or orange juice, which will only irritate the digestive tract further.

If any of the following symptoms occur, seek professional help:

1. Any abdominal pain that is persistent, especially if it is accompanied by tenderness, vomiting, diarrhea, or slightly raised temperature.
2. Persistent vomiting or diarrhea, especially if there is any presence of blood in the vomit or stool.
3. Signs of dehydration especially in the very young or elderly:

- Skin which loses elasticity: pinch a little skin on the back of the hand; if it doesn't spring back into shape quickly, check for other signs of dehydration.
- Lack of saliva or tears
- Sunken fontanel in babies (located at the crown of the head)
- Reduced urine output
- Sunken eyes

4. Any vomiting following a head injury.

CONSTIPATION

Type	General Indications	Worse From	Better From	Remedy
Constipation with hang-over	General irritability and headache accompany constipation. Lots of straining and fruitless urging. Never feels finished—incomplete passage of stool.	Eating Broken sleep Stimulants	Rest Sleep	**Nux Vomica** *Useful after abuse of drugs like painkillers and overuse of laxatives.*
Constipation without any urge to go	No desire to pass stool; total feeling of inactivity in bowel. Stool is uncomfortably large, very dark, dry, and painful to pass. Great thirst for cold drinks. Irritability and headache with constipation.	Heat Effort	Cold drinks Being still	**Byronia**
Constipation with soft, difficult stool	Difficulty passing sticky stools because of inactivity of the bowel. Stool will either be excessively soft, or hard and knotted. Itching and burning of anus with constipation.	Sitting still	Eating Warmth	**Alumina**

CONSTIPATION (cont.)

Type	General Indications	Worse From	Better From	Remedy
Constipation with anal fissure	Several days may go by with no urging, but once stool is passed it consists of small balls covered with mucus. Aching in rectum after passage of stool.	Cold Over-heating Before and after menstrual periods	Rest Open air	**Graphites**
Constipation away from home	Habitual constipation on vacation. Lots of fruitless urging with noisy wind and bloating. May feel anxiety about being constipated.	Travel Tight clothes Eating	Warm drinks	**Lycopodium**

Once the acute situation has been dealt with homeopathically, the following advice will help prevent the situation occurring again.

1. Have a good look at your diet, since in many cases
   constipation can be rectified or significantly
   improved by making certain dietary changes.
   Reduce foods that contain lots of white flour and
   sugar; also try to insure that dietary fat (butter,
   cheese, whole milk, and eggs) makes up no more
   than twenty percent of your total intake.

   It's best to put the emphasis on raw fruit and vegetables, whole-grain bread, and other foods naturally
   high in fiber, like lentils and beans.

   Try to also drink enough water. This sounds obvious, but many people do not realize that tea and coffee are no substitutes for water as a lubricant to the
   digestive system. Try to drink a minimum of four
   glasses of water a day and build up to eight.

2. It's best to avoid cooking with aluminum pans or
   using tea bags, which also use aluminum in the
   manufacturing process. Traces of aluminum in the
   diet can contribute to constipation, as well as a host
   of other problems including slow learning in the
   young, exacerbation of osteoporosis (brittle bones),
   and deterioration of the brain.

3. Always try to act on the urge to pass a stool — (provided of course it's socially acceptable!) Ignoring
   these important signals can be the first step to
   developing a problem with constipation.

4. It's best to avoid depending on laxatives to achieve a
   regular bowel movement, since the formation of this
   habit can lead to an ultimate aggravation of the
   problem by making the bowel become progressively
   more "lax." It is also very easy to get into a pattern
   of alternation of constipation with a form of diarrhea promoted by the overuse of laxatives: this can

lead in the end to problems of malabsorption where essential nutrients are not given the chance to be utilized by the body.

If you are concerned about any of the following symptoms, seek professional advice:

1. If for a period of time you experience a marked change in your bowel habit that is not attributable to a change in diet or routine.
2. Signs of blood in stool, especially if blood is dark in color.

HEMORRHOIDS

Type	General Indications	Worse From	Better From	Remedy
Hemorrhoids with sharp pains and swelling	Sensations as though rectum was full of sharp sticks after passing stool. Swollen sensation in rectum, and pains that persist for several hours.	Walking Bending	Cool	**Aesculus hippocastanum**
Bluish hemorrhoids with burning pains	Hemorrhoids that resemble a bunch of grapes in appearance. Bearing-down pains with burning, relieved by moving about.	Sitting	Bathing with cool water Moving about	**Aloe**
Hemorrhoids with shooting pains	Pains are stinging, burning, and shoot upward. Lots of itching in anus after passing stool.	Eating starch Warmth of bed	Resting	**Alumina**

HEMORRHOIDS (cont.)

Type	General Indications	Worse From	Better From	Remedy
Excessively sensitive hemorrhoids	Full sensation in hemorrhoids with constricted sensation in rectum. Bruised pains with sensations radiating up spine. Easy-bleeding hemorrhoids.	Exertion Alcohol and coffee	Resting Warmth	**Nux vomica**
Hemorrhoids with chronically inactive bowels	Painful sensitivity in rectum for hours after passing unusually large, hard, dry stool. No urge to go at all.	Warmth Moving	Resting Cool	**Bryonia**
Bleeding hemorrhoids	Sensations of bruised soreness with bleeding from the rectum. Hemorrhoids feel tense or bursting. Affected area feels swollen and inflamed.	Pressure Jarring Touch		**Hamamelis**

The pain and discomfort of hemorrhoids can be significantly eased by judicious use of homeopathic medicines. The following hints may also be useful in helping to deal with more deep-seated underlying factors that may be aggravating the condition:

1. Try to evaluate the quality of your diet, bearing in mind the advice already given in the Constipation section (p. 82). There is not much point in trying to ease the discomfort of hemorrhoids if your diet is causing habitual straining and constipation.
2. You may find a homeopathic ointment useful to soothe the painful area from without, as well as using homeopathic remedies internally. There are ointments on the market especially suited to this purpose, as well as a number of internal formulas. These should be available in health-food stores and pharmacies stocking homeopathic remedies.
3. It is also worth trying a warm bath before applying a soothing cream if hemorrhoids are inflamed and painful.

BEYOND THE IMMEDIATE PROBLEM: GENERAL ADVICE ON DIGESTION

All of us know by now about the value of exercise and its role in stress reduction, but perhaps fewer of us realize how helpful regular exercise can be to the healthy functioning of the digestive organs.

Apart from having a beneficial effect on stress levels (which has its own spin-off effect on digestion), regular exercise can help a great deal with a digestive problem like constipation. Lots of people suffer irregular bowel movements because of the lack of tone of their bowels, which can result from sitting in an office all day. This is a problem that can be further compounded by a bad diet, or just sheer lack of time for eating regular meals.

When choosing an exercise program, bear in mind that it needs to be one that suits your temperament. If exercise isn't enjoyable and fun, then the chances are that it will become a chore that only adds more stress to your life. Also try to aim for regularity rather than having long sessions of exercise at irregular intervals. It's more helpful to set aside twenty minutes every other day than to exercise furiously for an hour every two weeks.

Yoga can be very helpful in both aiding relaxation and improving muscle tone, which helps the digestive system to work more smoothly and effectively. More vigorous exercise, such as swimming or aerobics, especially when combined with stretching exercises, will also help combat constipation and generally make muscles more flexible as they become stronger. Bad posture can also contribute to many digestive problems, especially when it is compounded by a job that involves spending many hours a day hunched over a desk. Because so many of us today have jobs that are both sedentary and stressful, our digestive systems are often the first things to suffer. This makes the need for exercise even stronger, even if it only involves walking upstairs instead of automatically taking the elevator, or walking around the block to do some shopping instead of taking the car.

Therapies that look specifically at postural problems can also be something to consider if you have digestive problems, especially when these are combined with lower back pain. The Alexander technique, yoga, osteopathy, and chiropractic are all worth considering as possible sources of help.

Apart from looking at your diet and general life-style, it's worth taking a look at the problems associated with habitual use of antacids and laxatives.

Problems associated with the daily use of antacids include the syndrome *acid rebound,* which involves a

vicious circle of dilution of stomach acids, followed by the
stomach pumping in more acid to rectify the situation, as
a result of which more antacids are taken, and so on.
Some antacids also contain aluminum, which can contribute to constipation and has been linked to the development of presenile dementia; others contain bicarbonate of
soda, which leads to water retention, and should not be
used over long periods by those suffering from kidney
malfunction.

Laxatives cause their own problems when used on a
long-term basis. The main problem associated with regular use of laxatives (and this applies as much to a "natural" herbal laxative as to any other) is the tendency of the
bowel to lose the capacity to empty itself without the stimulation of a laxative. Once this happens, the problem of
being "hooked" on laxatives begins; this rather resembles
the vicious cycle I have described in my discussion of acid
rebound.

To end on an optimistic note, do not get discouraged if
all this seems foreign to you. Selecting the most appropriate remedy takes time, some effort, and a little bit of practice. However, once you become more familiar with the
remedies it gets progressively easier and you will become
more confident. But above all, once you achieve positive
results you will have the encouragement to continue.

5

Homeopathy and Emotional Symptoms

EMOTIONAL PROBLEMS

Short-term emotional problems, such as anxiety over a specific event or the transient depression that may follow an upsetting experience, are often seen as problems that do not require help from drugs, since they will often sort themselves out. If, on the other hand, the condition seems to be either so severe that it is incapacitating or it appears to be going on longer than one might reasonably expect, tranquilizers or antidepressants may well be suggested for short-term use. The rationale behind giving these drugs is that while they cannot remove the problems faced by the patient, they may give the person some space and distance within which to sort the problems out. Unfortunately, there are side effects to these drugs, which include drowsiness and fatigue, which can lead to impaired general functioning. Obviously, the long-term use of tranquilizers raises other more complex and controversial questions of physiological and psychological dependence.

Homeopathic Medicines and Emotional Problems

Since homeopathic theory starts from the premise that the mind and body are inextricably interlinked, there is nothing unusual about the use of homeopathic medicines for emotional disturbances. Because these medicines are understood to work by bringing the mind and body into an optimum state of equilibrium for the individual person, problems such as short-term anxiety need not pose an impossible problem for the prescriber. Homeopathic medicines used appropriately in cases of short-term anxiety can be very effective in calming the person down, without involving side-effects of drowsiness or fatigue. This also applies across the board to temporary sleep problems, grief, or shock.

Limitations of Self-Prescribing for Emotional Problems

While it is accurate to say that homeopathic medicines can be extremely effective in helping with emotional distress, a word of caution is needed. All of the tables below refer to emotional problems of recent onset in an otherwise healthy individual. If someone is suffering from long-term anxiety or depression, then it would be appropriate for that person to seek professional help from a qualified practitioner. This is needed for two reasons. Firstly, choosing an appropriate homeopathic medicine that covers the complexity of a case of long-standing emotional problems can be a subtle business that requires experience and professional expertise. Secondly, it is important to stress that on no account does the following section suggest that the homeopathic medicines below form substitutes for long-term use of drugs such as tranquilizers without the support of proper professional advice and treatment.

How to Select the Appropriate Homeopathic Medicine

If you have turned to this section of the book because you are suffering from anticipatory anxiety over a coming event, this is how you select your homeopathic remedy:

1. Turn to the table entitled Anticipatory Anxiety, and look down the left hand column entitled Type to identify which category your symptoms fall into. If, for example, you are normally outgoing and talkative, but as the day of an exam or stressful event approaches you become increasingly withdrawn and depressed, the chances are that the information given for "Anticipatory anxiety with withdrawn state of mind" is likely to be most appropriate.
2. Check the General Indications to see if these symptoms fit your own. If you feel exhausted with worry, droopy and trembly with nerves, and disinclined to make any physical or emotional effort, then it definitely looks like you are on the right track.
3. Finally check the Worse From and Better From columns to see if these also fit. Bear in mind that these two columns do not just refer to what makes your anxiety state better or worse, but also to what might make you feel better or worse generally. So, if you have definitely noticed that you feel worse in a stuffy room or dwelling on the coming event but feel much better being occupied in the open air, the chances are that Gelsemium is the most suitable remedy for you.
4. You will find some suggestions at the end of this section of the book for general ways of minimizing stress and anxiety through dietary measures, relaxation, and breathing techniques.

For information on how to take the appropriate remedy, see the section entitled How To Take Homeopathic Medicines (p. 8) in the chapter on practical homeopathy;

ANTICIPATORY ANXIETY

Type	General Indications	Worse From	Better From	Remedy
Anticipatory anxiety with lots of abdominal rumbling, gurgling, and wind	Anxiety often brought on by being required to speak in public. Although nervous beforehand, once begun, things go well. Anticipatory "nerves" involve much digestive disruption: lots of wind and bloating even after only a mouthful or two of food.	Being harried Being idle Stuffy rooms	Being occupied Open air	**Lycopodium**
Anticipatory anxiety with withdrawn state of mind	Exhaustion, droopiness and withdrawal with nervous states. Severe diarrhea with nervous worry. Apathy with disinclination for the slightest effort. Lots of trembling and internal feelings of weakness. Patient may feel subjectively cold.	Hot rooms Thinking of coming events	Open air Occupation Dietary stimulants from food or drinks	**Gelsemium**
Anticipatory anxiety with extreme agitation and desire to engage in conversation	Fear of a coming event with feelings of panic, palpitations, and tremor. Diarrhea may be brought on by general feelings of stress and tension. Restlessness from anxiety; possibly a craving for sugar to keep going, which aggravates the general condition. Symptoms worsen at night.	Stuffy rooms Sweets Waking	Open air	**Argenticum nit.**

ANTICIPATORY ANXIETY (cont.)

Type	General Indications	Worse From	Better From	Remedy
Anxiety with severe vomiting, diarrhea, and restlessness	Anxiety may manifest itself in an obsessional concern with tidiness even though the person may feel exhausted. Driven by restlessness to keep going. Extreme feelings of anxiety may lead to severe involvement of the digestive system including diarrhea and/or vomiting. May feel extremely chilly. Symptoms worsen at night.	Being alone Cold in any form	Warmth in any form Moving about Company	**Arsenicum album**
Anxiety with dependence on stimulants to get through the event	Very irritable and overwrought with feelings of anxiety. Sleep very disturbed, often the result of needing stimulants to keep going. May suffer from constipation and general digestive irritability. Symptoms worsen in early morning hours.	Being harried Being exposed to cold Stimulants	Resting undisturbed Warmth Napping	**Nux vomica**

exactly the same principles apply.

In addition to short-term use of the appropriate homeo-pathic medicine, the following suggestions may be helpful:

1. If you know that you have an event coming up that is likely to make you feel tense, try to arrange your commitments around that date so that they cause you the least amount of stress. In other words, if you know you have an exam or a driving test on a particular date, try to keep the day before it free, so that you have adequate time to mentally prepare for it.

2. Try to do something that you find restful on the day leading up to the event. This very much depends on you as an individual: some people might find a body massage or facial most soothing, while someone else might benefit more from a brisk walk, an exercise class, or something equally vigorous.

3. If you are having problems sleeping leading up to the event, avoid stimulating drinks such as strong tea or coffee before bed, or eating heavy meals before sleeping. A warm bath before bedtime using your favorite bath oil will be helpful. Generally speaking, a diet that is high in sugar, coffee, tea, or carbonated drinks is likely to make you feel on edge before a stressful event. It's a good idea to keep them to a minimum (but don't cut them out abruptly since this can lead to withdrawal symptoms), and concentrate on soothing drinks such as chamomile tea.

4. If you notice yourself breathing quickly and from your upper chest when feeling stressed or anxious, the advice at the end of this section on breathing and relaxation will be useful to you.

SHORT-TERM INSOMNIA

TYPE	GENERAL INDICATIONS	WORSE FROM	BETTER FROM	REMEDY
Sleeplessness from over-indulgence in food or alcohol	Strong mental irritability with sleeplessness. Lack of sleep may be the result of "burning the candle at both ends." Person may wake between 3:00 and 4:00 A.M., then fall asleep as it's time to get up.	Stimulants Being spoken to Cold drafts	Being left alone Warm drinks	**Nux vomica**
Sleeplessness with anxiety and strong restlessness	Person wakes between midnight and 2:00 A.M. Physical and mental restlessness and agitation. Feels much worse if cold, and generally better from warmth. Person may wake with a shock after falling asleep.	Being chilled Midnight to 2 A.M. Being over-tired	Warmth Warm drinks Company	**Arsenicum album**
Light sleeping after grief or bad news	Violent, spasmodic yawning with inability to get a decent night's sleep. Once sleep comes it may be disturbed by bad dreams or the same repetitive nightmare. Limbs jerk on going to sleep.	Emotional strain Yawning	Change in position Breathing deeply Being alone	**Ignatia**

Type	General Indications	Worse From	Better From	Remedy
Sleeplessness from muscular overexertion	Person tosses and turns in bed trying to find a comfortable spot. The bed generally feels too hard to be comfortable. Sleeplessness may follow a day in which muscles that are unused to working are overused. Physical restlessness.	Overexertion Being touched	Lying with head low	**Arnica**
Sleeplessness following a shock or disturbing experience	Panicky feelings with anxiety and restlessness. Person may feel convinced that they are going to die. Lots of tossing and turning, and nightmares when sleep does eventually come.	Fright Being in bed Being chilled	Fresh air Resting	**Aconitum**
Sleeplessness from aches and pains	Great despondency with inability to sleep. Aching in muscles and joints often responsible for lack of sleep. Pains may be triggered by exposure to damp cold. Restlessness with lots of tossing about and stretching. Symptoms worsen after midnght.	Damp and cold Resting	Warmth Hot bath Stretching	**Rhus tox.**

SHORT-TERM INSOMNIA (cont.)

Type	General Indications	Worse From	Better From	Remedy
Sleeplessness with persistent drowsiness and mind that won't switch off	Irritability with sleeplessness. The mind may be occupied with work or family worries. Dreams may also reflect these preoccupations. Sleep may be disturbed by recurrent thirst, and there may generally be a difficulty in getting to sleep before midnight.	Heat Being moved Early morning	Cool air Cold drinks Quiet	**Bryonia**

In addition to selecting the appropriate homeopathic medicine, the following advice will be helpful:

1. Try not to continue working until bedtime; try to do something that you find relaxing for an hour or two before you go to sleep.
2. Avoid heavy meals or stimulating drinks such as coffee before bed.
3. It's a good idea to have a regular pattern of exercise during the week so that your body and mind have a chance to deal with stresses and strains that naturally occur each day.
4. Have a warm bath before bedtime.
5. Try to eliminate light and noise from your room as much as possible, and make sure that it is neither too stuffy nor too cold.
6. If you cannot get to sleep, staying in bed and tossing and turning can make things worse. You could try getting up and making yourself a cup of chamomile tea (avoiding regular tea and coffee). Once you feel sleepy enough, you could go back to bed and try again.
7. The advice at the end of this section on breathing and relaxation will also help prepare you for sleep.
8. If you suspect that your sleeplessness is becoming a long-term problem, do seek professional advice rather than attempting to deal with it yourself. Insomnia would be seen by a homeopath as a condition needing constitutional treatment (treatment that is aimed at you as a whole person with the aim of improving your overall quality of health).

SUDDEN GRIEF AND EMOTIONAL SHOCK

TYPE	GENERAL INDICATIONS	WORSE FROM	BETTER FROM	REMEDY
Fearful reaction to bad news	Person is very frightened, restless, and fearful of death. Lots of agitation and may seem on the verge of collapse. Symptoms worsen at night.	Being touched Noise	Rest Open air	**Aconitum** *Often needed after witnessing or being directly involved in an accident.*
Shock symptoms with desire to be left alone	Symptoms accompany physical shock: person may claim that they are perfectly fine and push away those who are trying to help. May be morose mentally, but physically restless.	Touch Being approached After sleep	Lying with head low	**Arnica**
Strong agitation and violent weeping in grief that is not resolving itself	Violent, spasmadic weeping that may alternate with bouts of laughing. Lots of twitching and tremors, with constant sighing.	Touch Cold, open air	Being alone Eating Breathing deeply Near warmth	**Ignatia** *Very helpful where someone has news of a bereavement and feels they cannot cope without help.*

Type	General Indications	Worse From	Better From	Remedy
Grief which cannot be expressed	May want to cry, but feel they cannot in front of others so they hold back their emotions. Consolation makes everything worse because it's likely to bring tears to the surface. Generally feels relief from being alone.	Being consoled Company Noise	Being alone Rest Cool air	**Natrum mur.**
Suppressed anger from shock or bereavement	In grief may feel angry with themselves or with the person who has died for leaving them. Very physically and mentally sensitive. Symptoms worsen at night.	Being cold Any sensory stimulation	Warmth Rest	**Staphysagria** *Especially indicated where anger has been denied its natural expression.*
Grief or shock that leads to profound tearfulness and constant need for company	Strong need for sympathy and company, which helps. Very quickly moved to tears, which relieve. May have a fear of being left alone.	Stuffy rooms Resting Eating	Fresh, open air Sympathy A good cry	**Pulsatilla**

It is worth making the point that you should not feel compelled to give a homeopathic medicine to someone who is going through their reactions to grief and coping with them. In this situation, it is perfectly normal and necessary for someone to discharge the emotions relating to their grief. If however, they are clearly in need of extra help and support, or if the grieving process seems to be holding them back from getting on with their lives and not resolving itself, then short-term homeopathic prescribing can be immensely helpful.

In addition to choosing the most appropriate homeopathic medicine, the following suggestions may also be helpful:

1. Unfortunately, though many bereaved people find that in the first few days and weeks following the event they are surrounded by supportive and caring friends and relations, in the months that follow this cannot be maintained. Sadly, it often takes some months for someone to begin to accept that a death has taken place, and this is frequently the time when most support is needed but is not available. Close friends and family can be immensely important at this time in listening to how the bereaved person feels about their past and the future. This is likely to take time, but having someone to listen can help the person suffering their loss through this phase of their grief. If it looks like the grieving person needs a more objective ear, then counseling can be very helpful in supporting them and may often lead them to insights into their emotional responses.

2. If you have experienced a shock or bereavement, try not to push yourself too hard too soon. The body and mind are likely to need space within

which to recover, and this can take time. If this
need is ignored, it can have the effect of leaving
someone tired and exhausted for an extended period of time, when a shorter period of complete rest
at the appropriate time can have them back on their
feet sooner.

BEYOND HOMEOPATHY: GENERAL ADVICE

Breathing

Breathing is one of the basic functions that is essential
to preserving life, and yet it is astounding how little attention most of us pay to it. Because it can be classed as an
involuntary function many of us just take it for granted
that we may be concentrating on something totally different, and still we continue to take oxygen in and breathe
out carbon dioxide. And yet, breathing can be the key to
making us feel more or less stressed and anxious in a
potentially threatening situation. I have myself experienced the strain of being asked to reverse my car on my
driving test and having accomplished the task having the
examiner point out to me that it really was not necessary
to stop breathing in order to accomplish the maneuver
well! Holding one's breath or breathing rapidly and shal-
lowly from the upper chest are two of the commonest
ways of reacting to a situation that is fraught with anxiety.
Unfortunately, this only makes the situation worse, since
the balance of oxygen and carbon dioxide in the body is
disrupted, leading to more feelings of anxiety and stress,
which in turn cause more hyperventilation, and so the
vicious circle is perpetuated.

There is however, a positive side to all of this, since if
we know how to use our breathing most effectively in a
crisis, it is possible to break the vicious circle outlined

above and use the breath to help us relax, feel calmer, and more in control of the situation instead of the situation controlling us.

Next time you are feeling anxious or stressed, take a moment to observe how you are breathing. The chances are that you are breathing more rapidly than usual, and that the breaths you are taking in are very shallow. Also watch what part of your chest is doing all the work, and you will probably notice that all of the effort is coming from your upper chest. In order to help yourself feel more relaxed and calm, it is necessary to learn how to breathe using your diaphragm. At first it will probably feel a little strange, but once you have got the basic idea outlined below it will improve with time and practice.

Lie on your back with your knees bent and feet on the floor. Put one hand on your belly just above your navel and watch what happens as you breathe. In order to achieve diaphragmatic breathing, as you breathe in feel the hand resting on your belly being gently pushed up, and then feel it sinking down as you breathe out. The sequence you are trying to achieve on breathing in is first inflation of the belly followed by the chest, and on breathing out initial flattening of the chest followed by the belly. Try not to force this process too quickly as this will probably leave you just feeling tense and frustrated, but gently and slowly take a few breaths in and out becoming conscious of the action of your diaphragm.

If you feel a little light-headed just stop for a while and breathe normally; you have probably been breathing too deeply or too quickly or both. Once you feel back to normal, try again, always stopping if you need to. Once you have become familiar with this method, you can continue practicing sitting upright in a chair with your hand in the same position. Try to practice breathing this way for a few minutes each day, and you will soon find that you have got the basic idea. Once it has been grasped, you can use your breathing to help you in any stressful situation.

Relaxation

When we speak of relaxation, this need not be limited to specific relaxation techniques but can embrace a range of activities from listening to music, attending an exercise class, to having a warm bath. Whatever enables you to enjoy a sensation of relaxation and well-being is very important to identify, since it will play a major role in helping you relax when you are faced with a stressful event.

Perhaps the most important point about relaxing is that this is time that you are setting aside for yourself. If you are under strain it's very easy to forget that this is the very situation where you can benefit most from time spent in this way. Ironically, it's at times like these that most of us feel that either we're too hard-pushed to look after ourselves, or it's the last thing we feel like doing. Given this sort of situation, learning to value looking after yourself by taking just ten minutes or half an hour doing something that you enjoy, will leave you feeling refreshed and more able to cope. Above all, don't feel you have to fit in with other people's ideas of what constitutes a relaxing activity: find out what suits you as an individual, and most of all enjoy it.

Diet and Stress

There are certain foods that should be avoided in situations of general stress and anxiety, since they can have the effect of compounding the problem. These include foods that fit into the "quick-fix" category; in other words, foods that will stimulate you to activity in the short-term but leave a residual feeling of exhaustion. The main offenders are coffee, strong tea, carbonated drinks including caffeine and a high sugar content, chocolate, and refined cakes and cookies including a high proportion of sugar. If you are already feeling jittery about a coming event and are having trouble sleeping over it, depending on these foods will only kick your system into a higher state of arousal, making you feel more on edge. They also have the unfortunate effect of initially boosting your blood sugar level, which then drops dramatically, leaving you feeling tired, exhausted, and most likely irritable as well.

If you are feeling agitated and stressed, try altering the balance by cutting down on the foods mentioned above and replacing them with foods that avoid the peaks and valleys. These include fresh and dried fruit, teas that are known to have a calming effect such as chamomile, and as much freshly prepared food as possible concentrating on fish, poultry, and generous helpings of fresh vegetables. Try to have a regular eating pattern, rather than going long periods of time without eating and then snatching a snack when you can.

The general idea is to try and get the broad principles right, rather than feeling you have to get everything absolutely perfect at once, since this is only likely to lead to your feeling even more under stress and defeats the object of the exercise.

6

Homeopathy for Childhood Illnesses

CHILDHOOD INFECTIOUS ILLNESSES

Since the bulk of childhood infectious illnesses are viral in nature, there is little that the orthodox medical profession can offer as a way of dealing with the symptoms of such infections. Current measures available tend to concentrate either on ways of making the child comfortable, such as painkillers, or soothing topical preparations if there is a skin eruption once the infection has set in. The other increasingly promoted and controversial method of dealing with childhood infections is the use of immunization in the belief that it will act as a prophylactic agent, thus bypassing the susceptibility to disease. For a survey of books that deal with the complex and troubling issue of immunization, see Further Reading.

Homeopathic Medicines and Childhood Illness

Because homeopathic medicines are understood to work by stimulating the body's own defense mechanism to deal more effectively with disease, rather than attempting to find the specific agent that will fight the invading organism, infectious childhood illnesses pose no greater problem than any other disease to the homeopath. Infectious illnesses are viewed by many homeopaths as an opportunity for the young child's developing immune system to be given a "trial run," thus helping strengthen it for the future. When the appropriate homeopathic medicine is used to treat a child suffering from an infectious disease, pain will be eased, skin eruptions often cease to be as distressing, and the general course of the disease should be speeded up. The same also applies to the noninfectious childhood problems such as teething, since homeopathy has gained many supporters from desperate mothers who have found homeopathic medicines to be enormously speedy and effective in dealing with the general trauma of teething.

How to Select the Appropriate Homeopathic Medicine

If you have turned to this section of the book in order to find the appropriate homeopathic remedy to help a child who is suffering from the early stage of measles, this is how you set about it.

1. Turn to the table entitled Measles (p. 109) and look down the left-hand column entitled Type to identify which category your child's symptoms fall into. If your child is normally lively and outgoing but since being unwell is more withdrawn, tired, and apathetic, the chances are that the information given for "Early stage of illness with lethargy and great weariness" is likely to be most appropriate.

2. Check the General Indications to see if these symptoms fit your child's. If he or she is achy, shivery, and looks generally droopy and heavy-lidded, then

this confirms your selection. If not, try again.

3. Finally check the Worse From and Better From columns to see if these also fit. Do bear in mind that these two columns do not just refer to what makes your child's symptoms better or worse, but also to what might make him or her better or worse generally. So if you have noticed that he or she feels worse after making even the slightest effort but improves when exposed to fresh, open air, the chances are that Gelsemium will be the most helpful remedy.

4. Don't worry if *all* of the symptoms mentioned in connection with Gelsemium are not present in your child; remember that what you are looking for is the closest approximation to the overall picture presented by him or her. What you do need are some major keynotes to work with; in other words, one would not give Gelsemium to a child who did not seem shivery and withdrawn, or Belladonna to a child who was not flushed and agitated.

For information on how to take the appropriate remedy, see the section entitled How to Take Homeopathic Medicines (p. 8) in the chapter on practical homeopathy; exactly the same principles apply.

MEASLES

Type	General Indications	Worse From	Better From	Remedy
Early stage of illness with fearfulness and anxiety	Sudden onset of illness, often violent in intensity. Restlessness and fearfulness, which may be much worse at night. Catarrhal nasal discharge with very light-sensitive red eyes. Skin may feel burning as well as itchy. Hard-sounding, croupy cough. Symptoms worsen at night.	Warm rooms	Open air	**Aconitum**
Early stage of illness with hot, bright red, feverish skin	Very swift onset of symptoms. Skin is so hot and dry that one can feel heat radiating from it. Irritability and restlessness with illness. Drowsiness but inability to sleep. Throbbing head pains may accompany illness.	Light Noise Stimulants	Lying quietly propped up in bed	**Belladonna**
Early stage of illness with lethargy and great weariness	Slow onset of illness with alternating high temperature and chills and shivering. Drowsy, lethargic, and apathetic with drooping eyelids. Face may appear deep red and puffy. Aversion to moving even the head.	Making any effort	Open air Urinating	**Gelsemium**

MEASLES (cont.)

Type	General Indications	Worse From	Better From	Remedy
Measles with marked distressing eye symptoms	Lots of streaming discharges from the eyes with pronounced light sensitivity. Discharge from the eyes is burning and painful, while nasal discharge is bland. Nose and eye symptoms improve from exposure to open air. Hoarseness may accompany dry cough. Symptoms worsen in the evening hours.	Light Warmth Evening hours	Open air Blinking or wiping eyes	**Euphrasia**
Measles with swelling of the face, eyes, and eyelids	The rash may appear slowly with characteristic stinging pains. Rosy pink, puffy, itching eruptions that are relieved by cool bathing.	Heat Touch Sleep	Cool air and cool bathing	**Apis**
Later stage of measles once the rash has come out and fever has subsided	Dry mouth with no thirst. Cough alternates between dry at night and loose in the morning. Catarrh is bland, thick, and yellow-green in color. Rash is made worse by warmth and better by cool air. Ear pain may develop. Weepy with symptoms.	Stuffy rooms Rest Warmth Eating	Cool, open air Gentle motion	**Pulsatilla**

MEASLES (cont.)

Type	General Indications	Worse From	Better From	Remedy
Measles rash slow to develop with marked chest symptoms	Chesty cough causing pain in chest. Lots of tickling and irritation in larynx. Headache accompanies cough and feels much worse with any motion. Dry mouth with intense thirst for cold drinks. May be constipated and generally irritable with symptoms.	Any slight motion Sitting up Becoming heated Eating	Cool, open air Quiet Cold drinks	**Bryonia**

The following advice will be supportive of homeopathic treatment:

1. Encourage the child to drink as many fluids as possible. If he or she has a high temperature, they are unlikely to be hungry and it will not help to force food on them at this stage, but plenty of liquid is essential.
2. If there is light sensitivity, ensure that light is kept to a minimum by dimming lights or drawing curtains.

If any of the following occur, seek professional help:

1. Breathing difficulties.
2. Temperature registering over 104.
3. Measles in children under 6 months of age.
4. Earache.
5. Severe headache, lethargy, drowsiness or vomiting.
6. Bleeding from orifices or under the skin.
7. Cough is persistent for more than four days.
8. Any sign of eye infection.
9. Temperature doesn't resolve itself as the rash develops.

MUMPS

Type	General Indications	Worse From	Better From	Remedy
Rapid onset of mumps symptoms with terrific heat and redness	Marked restlessness with high temperature. Glands adjacent to the ears may look red and feel tender to touch. The right side may be particularly affected. Dry, burning throat with thirstlessness. Shooting pains in glands and throbbing headache.	Touch Light Noise	Lying down	**Belladonna**
Mumps with sensation of pressure and tension in glands	Hard, tense, stony feelings in glands adjacent to the earlobe and under the jaw. Dry throat with difficulty swallowing; pains shoot to the ears when attempting to swallow. Face and skin in general look pale (the opposite of patients requiring Belladonna). Symptoms worsen at night.	Cold and damp Warmth of bed Swallowing warm food or drink	Warmth in general	**Phytolacca**
Mumps with copious salivation and marked weakness	Marked weakness is followed by profuse perspiration. Dry mouth with free salivation, and marked dryness at the back of the throat. Tonsils may be swollen and jaws are likely to feel stiff. Speech may be difficult, with coating of the tongue.	Cold		**Jaborandi**

MUMPS (cont.)

Type	General Indications	Worse From	Better From	Remedy
Mumps with offensive breath and copious salivation and sweat	Sweating much worse with onset of night. Unpleasant, sweet metallic taste in the mouth with bad breath and swollen tongue. Symptoms worsen at night.	Extreme temperature changes Drafts Sweat	Rest	**Merc sol.** *Most likely to be indicated in the later stages of the illness, once the fever has peaked.*
Mumps with marked rosy, red swellings and heat sensitivity	Pains are stinging and feel much better with cool applications. Swellings are pronounced and look very puffy. Eyelids may look especially swollen. Constant fidgetiness and restlessness.	Warmth Lying down Sleep	Cool air Cool applications Change of position	**Apis**
Mumps with marked irritability and sensitivity to movement	Extreme sensitivity to motion, even of a single limb. Child is lethargic and wants to be left alone to lie still. Slow, insidious onset of illness with possible involvement of stubborn constipation. Marked thirst for large quantities of cold drinks, with dry lips.	Moving Heat Effort	Lying still Perspiration	**Bryonia**

MUMPS (cont.)

Type	General Indications	Worse From	Better From	Remedy
Mumps with pain that is much worse on the left side	Extreme sensitivity and swelling of the glands on the left side. Marked aversion to touch or pressure. Throbbing and constrictive pains. Swallowing is extremely painful and difficult.	Sleep Touch Empty swallowing Tight clothes around the neck	Open air Cold drinks Eating	**Lachesis**
Lingering mumps with involvement of breasts or testes in adults	Symptoms made generally worse by heat and better by open air. Child may be whiny, clingy, and generally attention-seeking. Dry mouth with coated tongue and lack of thirst. Symptoms worsen at night.	Stuffy rooms Lying down	Open air Gentle movement Consolation	**Pulsatilla**
Mumps symptoms that feel much worse from exposure to damp cold, and are much worse at night	Marked swelling of glands that may be much worse on the left than the right. Extreme restlessness and despondency at night with terrific sensitivity to cold and chilliness. Possible cold sores on the lips. Dreadful aching in the limbs, which rest aggravates. Symptoms worsen at night.	Cold and damp Rest	Heat Warm bathing Being wrapped up warmly	**Rhus tox.**

The following advice will be supportive of homeopathic treatment:

1. It is helpful to withhold acid drinks and spicy food from children when they have mumps since they will stimulate salivation, which will lead to increased pain.
2. Avoid letting children who are suffering from mumps come in contact with adults who have not contracted the disease, since the complications in adults can be very unpleasant. These include painful swelling of the testicles in males, and inflammation of the ovaries and/or the breasts in women.

If any of the following occur, seek professional help:

1. Stiff neck accompanied by weakness and/or headache or convulsions.
2. Inflammation of the breasts or testes in adults who have been in contact with the disease.
3. Difficulties with hearing or vision.
4. Abdominal pains, especially if accompanied by vomiting.

CHICKEN POX

Type	General Indications	Worse From	Better From	Remedy
Chicken pox with very itchy rash and extreme restlessness that is much worse at night	Dreadful itching, which is made much worse by scratching. Everything feels much worse at night, and there is likely to be much difficulty getting to sleep. Child is very chilly and cold-sensitive.	Scratching Cold	Warm bathing Moderate temperature	**Rhus tox.**
Chicken pox where the rash is very slow to develop	Large, slow-to-develop rash with accompanying rattling cough. Very bad temper with symptoms, with a tendency to moan and whine. Skin may be cold with a blue or pustular rash. Tongue may be white and thickly coated.	Cold Lying down	Cool air Bringing up phlegm	**Antimonium tart.**
Chicken pox with flushed, hot red skin and raised temperature	Very hot, bright red skin that feels very dry to the touch. Lots of drowsiness with inability to sleep. Throbbing headache with tendency to be sensitive to slightest stimulation.	Noise Bright light	Rest Warm room	**Belladonna**

CHICKEN POX (cont.)

Type	General Indications	Worse From	Better From	Remedy
Chicken pox with marked desire for warmth	Chill, restlessness, and anxiety. Eruptions look large and contain lots of pus. All symptoms generally seem worse at night.	Effort Cold	Warmth Lying with head raised	**Arsenicum album**
Chicken pox with swollen glands and offensive, copious sweat	Bad reaction to either strong heat or cold, and at night. Large eruptions with a lot of pus that may develop into sores. Sweat and breath are likely to be profuse and offensive. May complain of metallic taste in the mouth and increased salivation.	Heat Cold	Resting	**Merc sol.**
Chicken pox with low-grade fever and weepiness	Likely to be the later stages of chicken pox with swollen glands and lingering low-grade temperature. Child feels weepy and clingy and demands attention. Complains of chilliness, but feels better in open air. Symptoms worsen at night.	Stuffy rooms Resting Warmth	Open air Gentle motion Cool	**Pulsatilla**

The following measures are generally helpful in easing symptoms:

1. Try ways of preventing your child from scratching the eruptions, since this can lead to infection and scarring. One way of avoiding this is to trim the fingernails fairly short.
2. After bathing don't rub at the eruptions but try to pat them dry gently to avoid damaging the scabs.
3. If the skin is very itchy an oatmeal bath may be soothing, or try applying a diluted solution of Urtica urens tincture to the itchy areas of skin (available from homeopathic pharmacies).
4. If your child is not hungry don't feel compelled to push food on him or her. Meals should be kept as light and as easily digestible as possible.
5. Avoid using aspirin since it may be implicated in the development of Reye's syndrome (a serious, and often fatal illness characterized by high temperature, vomiting, and problems with liver and kidneys).

If any of the following occur, seek professional help:

1. Severe headache, marked weakness, convulsions, or stiff neck.
2. Vomiting or rapid, shallow respiration.
3. Bleeding under the skin.
4. Infection of skin eruption.
5. Chicken pox in a child of less than one year of age.

WHOOPING COUGH

Type	General Indications	Worse From	Better From	Remedy
Whooping cough with clammy, cold sweat	In bouts of coughing the child turns initially red and then becomes pale, cold and clammy. Strong desire for cool, fresh air. Burning sensations in chest with rawness of larynx and trachea. Cough is initially hard and dry, but lots of mucus is produced after the cough. Symptoms generally worsen at night.	Warmth Walking	Cool air Fanning	**Carbo veg.**
Whooping cough with wheezing, rattling cough	Child stiffens in a coughing bout and loses breath. Skin may take on a bluish shade in a coughing spasm. Episode of coughing ends in gagging and vomiting. Nosebleeds may accompany the cough.	Damp air Lying flat Motion	Open air Rest Cold drinks	**Ipecac**
Dry, metallic-sounding whooping cough with hoarseness	Severe bouts of coughing that follow each other in quick succession. Barking cough comes from deep in abdomen. The cough generally starts as soon as the child lies down. Symptoms generally worsen at night.	Resting Talking Warmth	Open air Being active	**Drosera**

WHOOPING COUGH (cont.)

Type	General Indications	Worse From	Better From	Remedy
Whooping cough that is worse in stuffy rooms	Episodes of coughing provoked by trying to clear throat of mucus. Coughing ends with vomiting of stringy mucus that hangs from the mouth.	Stuffy rooms Warmth	Sips of water	**Coccus cacti**
Whooping cough with sensations of smothering preceding bouts of coughing	Profuse nasal catarrh may accompany the cough, but the cough is likely to be dry. After coughing, vomiting of stringy mucus. Child feels too cold when uncovered, and too hot when covered.	Change of air Inhaling air Eating	Heat	**Corallium rubrum**
Whooping cough with easy expectoration	Chest feels sensitive during coughing bout. Dry, barking cough in cold air, becoming very loose when in a warm room. Choking sensation followed by vomiting.	Cold Drafts Being heated After exertion	Open air Moderate warmth	**Kali carb.**

TYPE	GENERAL INDICATIONS	WORSE FROM	BETTER FROM	REMEDY
Whooping cough with sore and bruised feelings in the chest	Cough aggravated during sleep and by exercise. Child may cry before cough sets in, anticipating the pain. Because of bruised feelings, child may hold the chest when coughing.	Damp cold Exertion	Resting	**Arnica**

See the general advice in the Cough section of Homeopathy for Sore Throats, Coughs, and Colds (p. 63). In addition, the following measures may be helpful:

1. Reassurance by a parent can do a lot to alleviate panic accompanying coughing bouts.
2. Small meals and drinks are best given just after a coughing bout.
3. Young babies can be assisted when coughing by holding them face down, with their bodies resting across your knees, while older children are helped by leaning forward while sitting.
4. Guard against dehydration by keeping fluid intake adequate.

For advice on when to seek help turn to the section on Coughs (p. 63), bearing in mind that special attention needs to be given to small babies since they are more vulnerable to complications.

EARACHE

Type	General Indications	Worse From	Better From	Remedy
Rapid onset of pain after exposure to dry, cold winds	Lots of anxiety and hypersensitivity to pain. Temperature may be high, with accompanying thirst and congested appearance. Noise causes great distress. Great restlessness. Symptoms worsen at night.	Noise Warm rooms	Sleep Open air	**Aconitum**
Violent sudden onset with very high temperature and redness	Tendency for the pain to lodge in the right side. Pains are violent, throbbing, and burning. Lots of irritability with the pains. Ear pain may extend to the neck, with accompanying sore throat and facial pain.	Stimulation Being touched Moving	Lying still Heat	**Belladonna**
Early stage of earache, which is milder than the indications in patients who require Aconitum or Belladonna	May be either flushed or pale with pain, or alternate between the two. Early stages of earache where mucus has not yet formed. Itching sensations in the ear with drawing pains.	Open air Exertion Noise	Gentle motion	**Ferrum phos.**

EARACHE (cont.)

Type	General Indications	Worse From	Better From	Remedy
Earache with extreme irritability and screaming	The pain puts the child in an extremely bad temper. Refuses to be comforted but may be soothed by being carried. Pains feel worse when child is bending over. May repeatedly try to cover ear for relief of pain.	Cold air Bending over	Warmth Being carried Being wrapped up	**Chamomilla**
Earache that accompanies the established stage of a cold	Nasal discharge that is bland, thick, and yellow-green in color. Earache may be severe, or cause little distress in the child. Child may feel chilly but reacts badly to warm rooms; may be uncharacteristically weepy or clingy. Symptoms worsen as evening approaches.	Stuffy rooms Warmth Rest	Cool Gentle motion	**Pulsatilla**
Earache that accompanies the middle stage of a cold, with thin discharge from the ear	Lots of weariness with cold and earache. Feels chilly and generally feels better when warmly wrapped up. Itching in the ear or stuffed-up feeling. Symptoms worsen at night.	Cold applications Moving Lying on painful side	Warmth Being well wrapped up	**Silica**

Type	General Indications	Worse From	Better From	Remedy
Earache with extreme cold sensitivity and irritability	Discharges are thick and yellow-colored. Cold makes the child very uncomfortable and bad-tempered, while wrapping up warm tends to be soothing. Pains are sticking and bursting. Symptoms worsen at night.	Cold drafts	Heat Being covered up snugly	**Hepar sulph.**
Earache with offensive, profuse sweating and discharges	Very bad reactions to extreme temperatures and to being in bed at night. Lots of salivation with possible metallic taste in mouth and flabby tongue. Possible glandular involvement.	Cold or heat Being in bed Sweating	Moderate temperatures	**Merc sol.**

The following measures will be helpful in minimizing pain and discomfort, and speeding up the healing process:

1. Drinking plenty of liquids will help flush toxins out of the body. Be careful to avoid milk and milk products, since these are thought to contribute to mucus formation.
2. As with any other infectious illness, it is very important to rest in order to allow the body to recover as quickly as possible.
3. A warm washcloth or heating pad could be applied to the ear if the pain responds well to heat.

If any of the following occur, seek professional help:

1. There is any weakness, lethargy, stiff neck, or severe headache.
2. A baby is pulling or rubbing its ear.
3. Any discharge in a child under the age of seven.
4. Any redness or tenderness in the bony area behind the ear.
5. Any sudden or noticeable decrease in hearing with or without pain.
6. Persistent discharge in an older child.

CROUP

Type	General Indications	Worse From	Better From	Remedy
Croup with extreme anxiety and restlessness	The early stage of croup with high temperature and restlessness. Cough is very dry, loud, and barking. The larynx may be sensitive to touch, and the child may grasp at the throat. Croup may follow soon after exposure to dry, cold air. Symptoms worsen at night.	Cold air Breathing in Touch Warm room	Open air Sweating	**Aconitum**
Croup with distinctive sound as though a saw were being drawn through dry wood	Wheezing and rasping with croup, with difficulty breathing between spasms. Cough sounds raw and dry with accompanying sense of suffocation. Not as anxious with fever as Aconitum.	Swallowing Exertion Talking Heat	Warm food Warm drinks Lying with head low	**Spongia** *If indicated, it follows Aconitum well.*
Croup with extreme cold sensitivity and irritability	Rattling cough with suffocative spells. Hoarse and wheezy with difficulty breathing. Very mentally and physically touchy and dissatisfied. Symptoms worsen in early morning.	Cold air Drafts	Moist heat Eating Warm wraps to head	**Hepar sulph.**

CROUP (cont.)

TYPE	GENERAL INDICATIONS	WORSE FROM	BETTER FROM	REMEDY
Croup that has passed the violent stage of recent onset but keeps recurring	Hoarseness and complete loss of voice may accompany croup. Tickly, dry cough, which responds temporarily to cold drinks. Lots of anxiety and restlessness accompany croup, with a strong desire for sympathy and attention. Symptoms worsen at night.	At night Cold air Touch	Sleep Eating Cold food and water, until they become warm in stomach	**Phosphorus**
Croup with metallic-sounding, brassy, hacking cough	Cough with thick yellow mucus discharged from the nose. Troublesome tickling in larynx with cough. Dry, burning, raw sensation in the throat. Hoarse voice, worse in the evening. Symptoms also worsen in morning. Generally indifferent with aversion to the slightest exertion.	Cold and damp	Heat Motion Bringing up phlegm Pressure	**Kali bichrom.**

Both keeping fluid intake up and putting the child in a steam-filled bathroom will help ease the condition. Reassurance is also needed for the child, since croup can be a very distressing experience.

If the child shows marked difficulty in breathing accompanied by drooling from the mouth, or if you are the least bit unsure about the seriousness of the condition, **seek professional help promptly**.

TEETHING

Type	General Indications	Worse From	Better From	Remedy
Teething that leads to terrific temper and screaming	Baby constantly puts fingers in mouth, seeking relief. Pain causes screaming and extreme irritability, which nothing seems to comfort. Baby may get to the point of screaming and hitting out at those around him/her; may only respond to being carried constantly. Symptoms worsen at night.	Heat Open air	Being rocked or carried	**Chamomilla**
Teething that causes great distress and weeping	Baby is more weepy than irritable with teething. May be woken from sleep with piercing cries of distress. Sighing, sobbing, and jerking may accompany teething symptoms.	After drinking	Biting Pressure	**Ignatia**
Teething with high temperature and extreme pain sensitivity	Baby is flushed, hot, and dry-skinned. Very sensitive to any sensual stimulation. Cheeks look red, hot, and swollen. Baby is very drowsy, but sleep is restless.	Noise Touch Jarring	Lying half propped up in bed	**Belladonna**

TEETHING (cont.)

Type	General Indications	Worse From	Better From	Remedy
Teething with whining and need for sympathy	Pains may be tearing and stitching, making the child weepy and in need of a lot of affection	Stuffy rooms Warm drinks	Cool, open air Cool drinks	**Pulsatilla**
Teething with severe inflammation of the gums	Spongy, inflamed gums that look very red. Child is likely to behave in a very agitated way when teething and is wakeful at night. Earache may accompany teething pains.	Cold At rest Lying down	Warmth Movement	**Kreosotum**
Teething with slow emergence of teeth and diarrhea	Very painful and slow teething. Colds and coughs may accompany teething process, as well as green-colored diarrhea. Closure of fontanel may be delayed.	Damp and cold	Warmth and dryness	**Calc. phos.**

Using a teething toy filled with cold water or a washcloth wrapped around some ice your child can bite on may do a lot to ease discomfort. Generally speaking, the most soothing things to gnaw on are soft, cool, and firm.

COLIC

Type	General Indications	Worse From	Better From	Remedy
Colic that is relieved by pressure	Colic leads to baby doubling up and screaming with pain. General restlessness, irritability, and anger. Pain in abdomen also feels better with warm applications. May have coated tongue.	At rest Motion Eating Drinking	Bending double Firm pressure Lying on stomach Passing wind	**Colocynthis**
Colic with violent temper and screaming relieved by being nursed	Baby moans and screams with pain. Very irritable, restless, and hard to please. May have accompanying diarrhea, which is green and offensive. Looks distended after eating.	Burping	Heat Being carried	**Chamomilla**
Colic that responds very well to warm applications	Sensitivity to cold drafts and general anxiety with pain. Lots of bloating with wind, leading to restless behavior. Clean tongue with colicky pains. Symptoms worsen at night.	Cold Being stretched out Motion	Doubling up Warmth Rubbing Belches	**Magnesia phos.**

COLIC (cont.)

Type	General Indications	Worse From	Better From	Remedy
Colic that is made much worse by movement	Irritability and crossness; the baby doesn't seem to know what it wants. May have constipation with colic and a marked thirst for cold drinks. Pains generally made worse by warm applications.	Moving Warmth Eating	Rest Firm pressure	**Bryonia**

If any of the following occur, seek professional help:

1. Any signs of dehydration:
   - Sunken fontanel (soft spot at the crown of the head)
   - Sunken eyes
   - Strong or decreased amount of urine passed
   - Dry mouth or eyes
   - Loss of skin tone
2. Pain in the abdomen appears to be severe.
3. Vomiting and diarrhea accompany colicky pain, or constipation.
4. Lethargy, screaming, or changed behavior with colicky pain.

BEYOND HOMEOPATHY: GENERAL ADVICE

In conclusion, it is worth mentioning that one should never be in doubt about calling on professional help if one is worried about a child's condition. Without being alarmist, it is worth bearing in mind that potentially serious childhood illnesses can develop rapidly and need identifying as quickly as possible. Children can get dramatically sick very quickly, so if there is any doubt in your mind, do get advice.

7

Questions and Answers About Homeopathic Treatment

How can I find a Homeopathic Practitioner?

You can obtain a directory of licensed health professionals who practice homeopathy in the United States from Homeopathic Educational Services and the National Center for Homeopathy. Although a directory is very useful in giving basic information about homeopathic practitioners in your area, I would strongly advise you to inquire whether any one you know has had successful homeopathic treatment: personal referral is probably the best way to locate a reputable practitioner. Obviously, this is not a foolproof method, since the relationship you develop with your homeopath will always be unique, and what is appropriate for one person may not be so successful for another. Nevertheless, if you have heard from a friend that the homeopath they consulted was professional, knowledgeable, sensitive, and perceptive to their individual needs, it would be well worth following this up with an inquiry.

This method is a useful way around the unconscious prejudice some people may have against lay practitioners who have not received conventional medical training; many of them are, in fact, extremely competent homeopaths. Obtaining the name of a homeopath by the referral method often bypasses the prejudice that some people may unwittingly have toward lay homeopaths, thinking that in order to have a responsible and well-qualified practitioner they must look for someone with conventional medical training. However, obtaining a recommendation from someone you know and whose opinion you trust will help you feel more confident about your choice of practitioner, whether he or she is an orthodox doctor or a lay homeopath.

Should I avoid orthodox drugs if I am taking homeopathic medicines?

Since homeopathic medicines are understood to work on the energy levels of the sick person they leave no traceable chemical constituents in the bloodstream or tissues. As a result, they are working on an entirely different level than orthodox drugs, which leave detectable traces in the body. Because of this major difference in approach and effect, there is little chance of the two medicines having an adverse interaction with each other and giving rise to undesirable side-effects.

Orthodox drugs that have a strong suppressive action, such as antibiotics, can interrupt the action of a homeopathic medicine, and patients who have had long courses of suppressive therapy may find that their systems take longer to respond to homeopathic treatment as a result. Viewed in this light, we can see that there is a basic incompatibility between orthodox and homeopathic medicines, which rests more on the level of the philosophy of illness than adverse biochemical interaction.

Are there certain foods I should avoid when taking homeo-pathic medicines?

Some foodstuffs are thought possibly to interfere with the action of homeopathic medicines: these include coffee, strong tea, and some herbal infusions such as peppermint (this also includes strong peppermint- or spearmint-flavored toothpaste). Always try to avoid taking a homeopathic remedy immediately after eating or drinking when there may be strong residual flavors in the mouth.

Can homeopathy help my sick pet?

Pets can benefit enormously from homeopathy for the whole range of conditions that affect large and small animals alike. To obtain homeopathic treatment for your pet, you need to contact the National Center for Homeopathy, Homeopathic Educational Services, or the American Holistic Veterinary Association, who can provide you with a list of vets who have undergone additional training in homeopathy. If you do not have a homeopathic vet in your area, inquire whether any of the vets on the list provide a telephone consultation service for routine conditions. There are a number of self-care manuals on the market for homeopathic treatment of acute conditions in animals, which can be helpful for obvious complaints, but as always, contact a professional if you suspect you are getting out of your depth.

Do homeopathic medicines lead to side-effects?

Because homeopathic medicines work by stimulating the body's own curative potential by boosting vital energy, side-effects produced by the medicines are not a problem, since there cannot be a buildup in the body. If the body is overstimulated by too frequent a repetition of a remedy, the original symptom for which the remedy was taken might get briefly worse. If this happens, all one has to do is to stop taking the remedy, and within a short space of time, things should return to where they were before the aggravation set in.

If one takes a remedy that is inappropriate for a relatively short space of time (up to three doses, an hour apart) all that is likely to happen is the disappointment of no response for the better. In this situation no harm has been done; just take another detailed look at the symptoms and see if another remedy is more strongly indicated.

Always remember that the most important thing to avoid is overfrequent administration of a homeopathic medicine. If it is working, always stop and wait. This is an indication that the body has been stimulated into action in a beneficial direction, and that it can cope very well by itself until the symptoms return. Once things start to slip back, you may repeat the remedy until improvement sets in again. If it looks like a remedy has stopped having a beneficial effect, take another look at the symptoms and see if another remedy is not more strongly indicated. If not, at this stage you may consider whether a stronger dose of the original remedy is called for.

Are there situations where homeopathy might not be of use?

Generally speaking, homeopathic prescribing is useful in any of the self-care situations outlined in this book. Categories of problems where homeopathic prescribing would be likely to produce disappointing results might include any situation where permanent tissue damage has occurred, problems that relate to a mechanical obstacle to recovery as in the case of displaced vertebrae, or cases where so much strong orthodox medication has been taken, it is difficult to differentiate between the patient's original symptoms and the side-effects of drug therapy.

Even in some of the situations outlined above, it is worth bearing in mind that homeopathic prescribing may still be very helpful in minimizing pain and distress as a useful adjunct to other therapies.

Can homeopathic medicines replace antibiotics?

There is no reason why homeopathic medicines cannot be prescribed in cases of bacterial infections with effective results, provided the prescribing is accurate and competent. As we have stated earlier in this book, homeopathic medicines are capable of aiding the body in its fight against the range of bacterial or viral infections by stimulating the body's own defense mechanism. Clearly, the results obtained will depend very much on the experience and skill of the prescriber, but it is very helpful to use the indicated homeopathic remedy as the first resort, keeping the antibiotic in reserve if the expected improvement is not forthcoming.

It is obvious that a professional practitioner is more likely to be able to prescribe with the accuracy needed to institute a healing response in the minimum amount of time. It is also true that if a homeopathic practitioner is professional in their approach to clinical signs and symptoms, they will pick up indications that suggest that improvement is not forthcoming and that the situation is worsening. It must be said effective homeopathic treatment in skilled hands can avoid the overuse of antibiotics, leaving the latter as a last-ditch strategy for those situations that are sluggish in response to more holistic measures.

As always, never proceed with self-help prescribing if you feel the situation is deteriorating and you are feeling anxious about it. Do get professional help and advice rather than feeling you must soldier on by yourself.

Should I have my child immunized if he or she is receiving homeopathic treatment?

The issue of immunization is one that is fraught with controversy because of the emotive nature of the debate with regard to children. Many homeopaths will present a strong argument against immunization, arguing that vaccines do not provide long-term immunity to the diseases being vaccinated for, and that there may be long-term side-effects following immunization including susceptibility to recurrent ear infections, allergic reactions, and skin problems. Homeopaths also draw attention to the different processes involved in acquiring a natural immunity to infectious disease when compared with the immune response engendered by immunization. Infection of one child from another who has a childhood disease such as measles involves a systemic response in the infected child over an extended period of time; by the stage the symptoms of high temperature, aching, and rash have appeared the immune system has begun to produce antibodies against the virus. Injection of a vaccine into the bloodstream provokes only an antibody response rather than mobilizing a systemic inflammatory reaction and may leave residual viral elements in the body for an extended period of time.

Clearly, the whole issue of immunizing—or not immunizing—your child is one that can be fraught with guilt, confusion, and anxiety. If you consult a homoeopath about yourself or your child, I would suggest you discuss the issue with them in detail, especially with regard to what homeopathic measures can be taken in the situation of a child developing one of the infectious childhood illnesses. There are also a growing number of books and articles available on this subject, which I would suggest you read before making an informed decision either way. The material included in these publications should make it easier for you to have a useful discussion with your family doctor about this very complex issue. If you would like more information on this subject turn to Further Reading.

Can I use other alternative therapies if I am receiving homeopathic treatment?

Most therapies that fall into the "alternative" category, such as massage, osteopathy, chiropractic, reflexology, or autogenic training, can be used side by side with homeopathy. Any therapy that has at its heart the aim of helping the individual achieve the maximum amount of balance and harmony in mind and body has a very similar aim to homeopathy as a system of healing. Yoga and the Alexander technique may both be helpful in teaching the homeopathic patient more about the way they move and respond to stress, while basic relaxation techniques can do a great deal to help someone come to terms with how they deal with the amount of mental and emotional strain they may have in their lives. Some homeopaths suggest that acupuncture, although it has much in common with homeopathy as a holistic system of medicine, may not work easily in harmony with homeopathic treatment. In these cases, it is often suggested that the patient concentrate on one of these two therapies for a set period of time to assess the benefits of each independently.

Once you begin to experience homeopathy as a system of healing for yourself and others, it is often noticeable that a natural examination of life-style and diet begins. This is a very positive development, since there is little point in substituting homeopathic medicines for orthodox drugs if there is an underlying dietary factor that is leading to the problems as in the case of excess drinking or a highly-indigestible diet. This most emphatically does not mean that you need to become a strict vegetarian, or give up alcohol or other foods that give pleasure in modera-

tion: a harsh or puritan approach will not lead to a sense
of balance either. But as you become more familiar with
what leads your body to experience a sense of enhanced
well-being and what does the reverse, the chances are that
you will want to maximize your optimum level of good
health by supporting your body, rather than fighting
against it.

Appendix i

Remedy Keynotes

ACONITUM

- Most likely to be of use in the first stages of illness rather than established stages.
- Strong affinity for respiratory organs.
- Conditions of sudden, violent onset.
- Extreme anxiety with specific fear of death.
- Conditions often follow from exposure to dry, cold winds.
- Strong intolerance of pain with extreme restlessness and anxiety.
- Symptoms worsen at night.

Worse From:
Warm rooms

Better From:
Open air

APIS

- Often indicated in allergic skin reactions.
- Red, puffy swellings that appear with rapidity.
- Puffy swellings may appear around the eyes, mouth, or in the throat.
- Stinging, burning pains that are relieved by cold.
- Conditions may follow a rash that has disappeared or failed to appear.
- Scanty urination and discharges.

Worse From:
Heat

Better From:
Cold air and applications

ARNICA

- Indicated in the first stage of trauma, shock, and bruising following accidents.
- Bruised and aching sensations with extreme restlessness.
- Weariness, soreness, and prostration.
- Cannot get comfortable in any position, especially in bed.
- Strong aversion to being touched; may fear the approach of anyone.
- Patients claim that they do not need attention, all they want is to be left alone.

Worse From:
Touch
Heat
Rest

Better From:
Lying with head low

ARSENICUM ALBUM

- Strong affinity for organs of digestion and respiration.
- Pains that are generally burning: throat, stomach, skin, etc.
- Acrid, burning, scanty discharges.
- Chilliness and prostration by illness.
- Marked anxiety and restlessness, which is aggravated at night.
- Wants air but is sensitive to cold in general.
- Peculiar symptom of burning pains relieved by warmth.
- Most symptoms are relieved by keeping warm, except for head symptoms, which are improved by cool air.
- Symptoms worsen at night, especially after midnight.

Worse From:
Cold (except for head)
Sight or smell of food
Being alone

Better From:
Warmth
Sips of hot drinks
Lying propped up in bed

BELLADONNA

- Indicated in early stage of illness with sudden, violent onset.

- Bright red, dry skin with bounding pulse.
- Sensitivity to external impressions: light and noise, etc.
- Agitation and irritability.
- May be delirious with dilated pupils.
- Symptoms occur largely on the right side: earache, sore throat, etc.
- Restless sleep with muscular twitching.

Worse From:
Noise
Light
Lying down
Moving

Better From:
Sitting up in bed in a darkened room
Keeping still in a warm room

BRYONIA

- Slow-developing symptoms.
- Dryness of mucous membranes, stool, cough, etc.
- Headache may accompany most ailments.
- Irritable and touchy with illness: just wants to be left alone.
- Moving makes most symptoms worse.
- Instinctive desire to press the affected part in order to hold it still, especially the chest and the head.
- Strong aversion to warmth and a general desire for cool.
- Thirst is very marked for large quantities of cold water.

Worse From:
Movement
Heat
Eating

Better From:
Cold
Keeping still
Pressure

CARBO VEG.

- Air hunger with collapse.
- Skin is pale, clammy, and tinged with blue.
- Chilly in general, but wants to be uncovered when feeling cold.
- Internal burning with external coldness.
- Lots of flatulence with heavy sensations in stomach.

Worse From:
Warmth
Lying down
Fatty food

Better From:
Being fanned
Belching

GELSEMIUM

- Complaints that develop slowly over a period of days.
- Aching, weary, and exhausted sensations.
- Shivers run up and down spine.
- Everything feels heavy, especially the eyelids, which look droopy.
- Indifference to anything due to lack of energy.
- Congestive sensations, especially in the head.
- Dark red, deeply flushed face.
- Lethargy, incoherence, and forgetfulness.
- Very chilly with cold extremities.

Worse From:
   Exertion
   Lying with head low

Better From:
   Bending forward
   Open air
   Sitting still propped up by pillows

HEPAR SULPH.

- Sensitivity to cold and drafts of cold air.
- Peculiar and characteristic sensation of a sticking pain in the throat as though a fish bone were lodged there.
- Marked irritability, chilliness, and hypersensitivity.
- Pains are very severe, sharp, and sticking.
- Lots of catarrh and a tendency to suppuration.
- Thick, yellow, offensive-smelling discharges.
- Night sweats that give no relief.

Worse From:
   Cold
   Touch
   Exertion

Better From:
   Wet weather
   Warmth
   Wrapping up warmly

HYPERICUM

- Marked affinity for injury to areas rich in nerve supply, e.g., fingers, toes, base of spine.

- Often indicated in puncture wounds with shooting pains.
- Useful for residual nerve pain following dental work.
- Promotes healing of jagged lacerations.

Worse From:
Touch
Cold

Better From:
Bending head back

IGNATIA

- The main remedy to think of in cases of emotional shock and grief.
- Muscular spasms especially affecting the digestive tract giving rise to hiccupping.
- Repeated sighing.
- Uncontrollable weeping.
- Contradictory symptoms, e.g., indigestion relieved by eating.
- Upredictability of moods: moves quickly from one extreme to another.

Worse From:
Emotional strain
Strong odors
Tobacco, coffee, and alcohol

Better From:
Warmth
Distraction
Eating

LACHESIS

- Affinity for the throat, and left-sided complaints.
- Disturbances of the circulation, leading to a bluish-purple tinge to the skin.
- All symptoms are much worse from sleep.
- Nerves and the senses in general are likely to be overwrought.
- Throat is very sensitive to touch.
- Strong suffocative sensations: must rush for air.
- Tendency to glandular swelling and sensitivity of the neck.

Worse From:
Sleep
Touch
Becoming warm

Better From:
Onset of discharge
Fresh air
Removing any constricting garment from around the neck

LEDUM

- Strong affinity for injured joints, fibrous tissue, and tendons.
- Affinity for puncture wounds.
- Tendency for affected part to feel cold to the touch.
- Affected area looks red and swollen.
- Pains are throbbing.

Worse From:
Warmth
Heat of the bed

Better From:
Cold applications

LYCOPODIUM

- Symptoms have a marked tendency to move from right to left.
- Lots of digestive disturbance: belching, rumbling, gurgling, and bloating.
- Marked aggravation between 4:00 and 8:00 P.M.
- Generally chilly and better from warmth, except for head symptoms which are better from cold.
- Throat symptoms, relieved by warm drinks.
- Periodic headaches associated with digestive disturbance.
- Tendency to diarrhea often combined with anxiety.
- Burning pains, especially in the digestive tract.
- Symptoms worsen in late afternoon.

Worse From:
Cold drinks
Cold air
Overexertion

Better From:
Warmth
Warm drinks
Open air

MERCURIUS SOLUBILIS

- Discharges that are copious and offensive.
- Marked swelling and flabbiness of tongue, which takes imprint of teeth.
- Saliva much increased and has metallic taste.
- Tendency to glandular swelling and aching.

- Night sweats very marked with offensive odor.
- Marked tendency for ulcers, abscesses, boils, and pus formation in general.
- Terrific sensitivity to extremes of temperature.
- Most symptoms feel worse from becoming warm in bed.
- Symptoms worsen at night

Worse From:
Sweating
Heat of the bed
Extreme temperature changes

Better From:
Resting
Moderate temperatures

NATRUM MUR.

- Dryness of mucous membranes.
- Nasal discharge alternates between copious, clear mucus, and a thicker, more scanty discharge like egg white.
- Stubborn constipation.
- Skin is generally cracked and dry, especially around the lips.
- Chronic tendency to cold sores.
- Marked emotional disturbance, which cannot be relieved.
- Desire to cry, but cannot, especially in company.
- Symptoms may be brought on by suppressed reactions to grief or reprimand.
- Lots of allergic symptoms: itching skin, sneezing, watery eyes, etc.

Worse From:
Consolation

Noise
Talking

Better From:
Being left alone
Skipping meals
Open air

NUX VOMICA

- Often indicated for symptoms that follow "burning the candle at both ends" or general overindulgence in food and alcohol.
- Oversensitivity is marked on both mental and physical levels.
- Headaches accompany most symptoms, especially constipation.
- With constipation there is a marked symptom of incomplete evacuation of stool with a sensation as though something had been left behind.
- May feel relief would be obtained by vomiting but must strain to do it.
- Generally very chilly, and feels much worse for being exposed to drafts of cold air.
- Very irritable, snappy, and argumentative.
- Generally much better if person is left alone.

Worse From:
Being spoken to
Any form of stimulation
Eating
Being exposed to a chilly, drafty environment

Better From:
Having a nap
Being left undisturbed
Avoiding food

PHOSPHORUS

- Marked tendency to glandular swellings and recurrent sore throats.
- Tightness and oppression of chest with irritating, tickly coughs.
- Catarrh is often yellow.
- Hoarseness that gets worse as the evening goes on.
- General tendency to flushes of heat.
- Marked thirst for cold drinks.
- Terrific sensitivity to atmospheric changes, e.g., headaches may warn of an approaching thunderstorm.
- Very mentally and physically reactive to stimuli.
- Easily exhausted.
- Symptoms worsen in the evening.

Worse From:
Physical or mental exertion
Warm food or drink
In a thunderstorm

Better From:
Cold food and drink until it gets warmed in the stomach
Being touched and reassured

PULSATILLA

- Often indicated in the later, established stage of illness.
- Very chilly but feels much better in fresh, open air.
- Changeability of symptoms on both emotional and physical levels.
- Discharges from mucous membranes may be thick, green, and bland.
- Weepiness accompanies most symptoms with a strong need for sympathy.

- Dry mouth with no thirst.
- Sensitivity to rich and fatty foods, which leads to indigestion.

Worse From:
Stuffy rooms
Resting
Eating

Better From:
Gentle exercise
Open, fresh air
Sympathy

RHUS TOX.

- Aching limbs and joints that are relieved by gentle exercise but feel worse from overexertion.
- Most symptoms are much worse at night, especially in bed.
- Very sensitive to cold and damp.
- Pains are relieved by a warm bath.
- Very restless and despondent with pain.
- Aching in bones with fevers and influenza.
- Skin can be intolerably itchy, red, and blistered.
- Symptoms worsen at night.

Worse From:
Keeping still
Overexertion
Cold, wet weather

Better From:
Gentle movement
Warmth
Dry weather

Appendix ii

Homeopathic Remedies and Their Abbreviations

Remedy	*Abbreviated Name*
Aconitum napellus	Aconitum
Aesculus hippocastanum	Aesculus
Allium cepa	
Aloe socotrina	Aloe
Alumina	
Antimonium crudum	Antimonium crud.
Antimonium tartaricum	Antimonium tart.
Apis mellifica	Apis
Argenticum nitricum	Argenticum nit.
Arnica montana	Arnica
Arsenicum album	Arsenicum
Belladonna	
Bellis perennis	Bellis
Bryonia alba	Bryonia
Calcarea carbonica	Calcera carb.
Calcarea phosphorica	Calcera phos.
Calendula officinalis	Calendula
Cantharis	
Carbo vegetabilis	Carbo veg.
Causticum	
Chamomilla	
Coccus cacti	Coccus
Colocynthis	
Corallium rubrum	Corallium
Cuprum metallicum	Cuprum
Drosera rotundifolia	Drosera
Dulcamara	
Eupatorium perfoliatum	Eupatorium
Euphrasia	

Remedy	*Abbreviated Name*
Ferrum metallicum	Ferrum met.
Ferrum phosphoricum	Ferrum phos.
Gelsemium sempervirens	Gelsemium
Glonoinum	
Graphites	
Hamamelis virginica	Hamamelis
Hepar sulphuris calcareum	Hepar sulph.
Hypericum perfoliatum	Hypericum
Ignatia amara	Ignatia
Ipecacuanha	Ipecac
Jaborandi	
Kali bichromium	Kali bichrom.
Kali carbonicum	Kali carb.
Kerosotum	
Lachesis	
Ledum palustre	Ledum
Lycopodium	
Magnesia phosphorica	Magnesia phos.
Mercurius solubilis	Merc sol.
Natrum muriaticum	Natrum mur.
Nux vomica	Nux vom.
Phosphorus	Phos.
Phytolacca decandra	Phytolacca
Podophyllum pelatum	Podophyllum
Pulsatilla nigricans	Pulsatilla
Pyrogenium	Pyrogen.
Rhus toxicodendron	Rhus tox.
Rumex crispus	Rumex
Ruta graveolens	Ruta
Sabadilla officinarum	Sabadilla
Sanguinaria	
Sepia	
Silica	
Spongia tosta	Spongia
Staphysagria	
Sulphur	Sulph.
Symphytum officinale	Symphytum
Thuja occidentalis	Thuja
Urtica urens	Urtica
Veratrum album	Veratrum alb.

Further Reading

SPECIFIC BOOKS ON SELF-CARE

The Complete Homeopathy Handbook: A Guide to Everyday Health Care. Miranda Castro. New York: St. Martin's Press, 1990.

Everybody's Guide to Homeopathic Medicines: Taking Care of Yourself and Your Family with Safe and Effective Remedies. Stephen Cummings and Dana Ullman. Los Angeles: Tarcher/Perigee, 1991.

Family Guide to Homeopathy. Barry Rose. Berkeley: Ten Speed Press, 1993.

The Family Guide to Homeopathy: The Safe Form of Medicine for the Future. Dr. Andrew Lockie. New York: Fireside, 1989.

The Homeopathic Emergency Guide. Tom Kruzel. Berkeley: North Atlantic Books, 1992.

Homeopathic Medicine at Home. Maesimund Panos and Jane Heimlich. Los Angeles: Tarcher/Perigee, 1980.

Homeopathic Medicines for Children and Infants. Dana Ullman. Los Angeles: Tarcher/Perigee, 1992.

Homoeopathy for Mother and Baby: Pregnancy, Birth and the Post-Natal Year. Miranda Castro. London: Macmillan, 1992.

156

Homeopathic Medicines for Pregnancy and Childbirth. Richard Moskowitz. Berkeley: North Atlantic Books, 1992.

Sports and Exercise Injuries. Stephen Subotnick, Berkeley: North Atlantic Books, 1991.

The World Traveller's Manual of Homoeopathy. Colin Lessel. Essex, England: C.W. Daniel, 1992.

GENERAL INTRODUCTIONS TO HOMEOPATHY

Discovering Homeopathy: Medicine for the 21st Century. Dana Ullman. Berkeley: North Atlantic Books, 1991.

Homeopathy: An Introduction for Beginners and Skeptics. Richard Grossinger. Berkeley: North Atlantic Books, 1994.

Homeopathy, Medicine for the New Man. George Vithoulkas. New York: Arco, 1979.

If you wish to go beyond a general introduction to homeopathy and obtain more specific information on the theory and philosophy of homeopathy as a medical science, the following books will be of interest:

The Handbook of Homeopathy. Gerald Koehler. Rochester, Vt.: Healing Arts, 1987.

Homoeopathic Science and Modern Medicine: The Physics of Healing With Microdoses. Harris Coulter. Berkeley: North Atlantic Books, 1980.

The Science of Homeopathy. George Vithoulkas. New York: Grove Press, 1980.

The Spirit of Homoeopathy. Rajan Sankaran. Bombay: Homoeopathic Medical Publishers, 1991.

Books that provide an overview of the historical development of homoeopathy include:

Divided Legacy: The Conflict Between Homoeopathy and the American Medical Association. Harris Coulter. Berkeley: North Atlantic Books, 1982.

A Homeopathic Love Story. Rima Handley. Berkeley: North Atlantic Books, 1990.

IMMUNIZATION

The following provide a survey of the arguments for and against immunization:

The Immunization Decision: A Guide for Parents. Dr. Randall Neustaedter. Berkeley: North Atlantic Books, 1990.

Vaccination and Immunization: Dangers, Delusions and Alternatives. Leon Chaitow. Essex, England: C.W. Daniel, 1987.

VETERINARY HOMEOPATHY

Cats: Homoeopathic Remedies. George MacLeod. Essex, England: C.W. Daniel, 1990.

Dogs: Homoeopathic Remedies. George MacLeod. Essex, England: C.W. Daniel, 1983.

The Homoeopathic Treatment of Small Animals: Principles and Practice. Christopher Day. London: Wigmore Publications Ltd., 1984.

Homeopathic Resources

HOMEOPATHIC ORGANIZATIONS

American Institute of Homeopathy
1585 Glencoe Street #44
Denver, CO 80220

International Foundation for Homeopathy
2366 Eastlake Avenue East # 301
Seattle, WA 98102

Foundation for Homeopathic Education and Research
2124 Kittredge Street
Berkeley, CA 94704

Homeopathic Academy of Naturopathic Physicians
14653 South Graves Road
Mulino, OR 97042

National Center for Homeopathy
801 North Fairfax # 306
Alexandria, VA 22314

SOURCES OF HOMEOPATHIC MEDICINES

Biological Homeopathic Industries
11600 Cochiti S.E.
Albuquerque, NM 87123

Boericke and Tafel
2381 Circadian Way
Santa Rosa, CA 95407

Boiron-Bornemann, Inc.
1208 Amosland Road
Norwood, PA 19074

also: 98c West Cochran
Simi Valley, CA 93065

Dolisos
3014 Rigel
Las Vegas, NV 89102

Homeopathic Educational Services
2124 Kittredge Street
Berkeley, CA 94704

Luyties Pharmacal
4200 Laclede Avenue
St. Louis MO 63108

Standard Homeopathic Company
204–210 West 131st Street
Los Angeles, CA 90061

SOURCES OF HOMEOPATHIC BOOKS, TAPES, AND SOFTWARE

Homeopathic Educational Services
2124 Kittredge Street
Berkeley, CA 94704

Veterinary Information

The American Holistic Veterinary Association
2214 Emmorton Road
Bel Air, MD 21014

As a practicing homeopath, **Beth MacEoin** MNCHM, RS Hom., brings her professional experience to this invaluable family guide.